Contents

Foreword

Why bother to write for a scientific or medical journal? Why not go to a football match, learn the oboe, or become a 'wall of death' rider instead? Tim Albert tells readers in this excellent book 'to be absolutely clear why you want to be published'. If you decide that you do and are overawed then Tim's book will be a huge help. It will motivate, prompt, guide, nudge, amuse and even console you as you make the journey to the front page of *The Lancet* – or the *Transactions of the Barsetshire Urological and Literary Society*. And if you decide you don't care about being published, Tim suggests you go fishing. That's wisdom.

The first reason to want to be published is because you have an earth shattering discovery to announce. If you have worked out the structure of DNA or discovered the cure for Alzheimer's disease, then you have no need to worry about being published. Increasingly, people send for CNN instead of publishing a paper, but if you do decide to write a paper then it's bound to be published – unless it's so opaque that the editors can't work out what on earth you've done. There are such papers.

Often your piece of research seems to you as important as working out the structure of DNA. Just as we think our small children are the smartest we've ever met, so we lose perspective over our research. The vast majority of readers of this book will never win a Nobel prize, and so you need to work hard at getting your paper published. This book will help.

Maybe you want to get published not because you have

research results to announce but because you have 'something to say'. Perhaps you are a specialist worked into a frenzy by the mistakes that generalists make when referring patients to you. You want to set them straight. This is a good motivation to publish, but you may find it hard. You may sound to the editors like a fanatic (perhaps you are). Editors like passion (or at least I do) because readers like passion. The problem with passion in writing is to contain it. Uncontained passion leads to boring, unstructured, incomprehensible writing. This book will help you avoid that trap.

You may want to get published to be part of the medical and scientific debate. That's a good reason but be prepared for the consequences, one of which is that nobody pays any attention to what you publish. Nobody mentions it, nobody responds. Another possible consequence (which just happened to me) is that you receive 26 letters, two of them insisting that you be sacked. Response is hard to predict.

And yes, it is reasonable to want to publish because you want to get on in your career. Tim says: 'There is no need to be ashamed. This is a fact of contemporary life, and if you don't compete you will lose out. Whether you approve of it or not is irrelevant?' Amen.

Finally, you should publish to keep me in a job. Editors may fall victim to their own pomposity and power, but without authors there would be no editors. We need you more than you need us.

RICHARD SMITH
London
August 1996

Preface to the second edition

One of the few sad things about authorship is that the world doesn't stop changing just because your book is finished. I am therefore grateful to Radcliffe Medical Press for giving me the opportunity to produce a second edition of this one so soon after the first.

It was encouraging to realise that the 10 steps of writing a scientific paper still stand, as does the overall approach, which is to persuade and encourage would-be writers to write, and not frighten them with hundreds of instructions. As far as I can tell, this remains an unusual approach.

I have made four specific changes. In the first edition, much of the advice was based on an analysis of 89 articles published in the *BMJ*. I have extended this research to 300 articles in six different journals, and this has brought out some unexpected differences between, for instance, general and specialist, European and US journals. Second, I have reviewed all the recommendations in the *Bookchoice* sections, adding some new works, recommending the second editions of others, and sticking to some trusted favourites. Third, I have changed my advice in a few places, specifically in the sections on structure and free writing. Finally, I have added a new introduction, which deals with the extraordinary changes taking place in electronic publishing and raises the question: are the skills taught in this book actually of any use?

I have also taken the opportunity to erase some of those awful phrases that you come across when you re-read your own work, and wonder how you could have put them there in the first place. I have also updated in a number of areas, for example taking into account the latest impact factors and incorporating the most recent guidelines from the Vancouver Group.

Apart from repeating my thanks to those who have helped in the past, I would like to thank Heidi Allen for inviting me to prepare a second edition, Kathryn Hampson for her help with the research and my wife Barbara for reading the manuscript so carefully. I would like to dedicate this edition to the memory of my friend Bill Whimster, who died shortly after the first edition was published. He and I taught and learnt together for several years, and his absence has underlined how much I owe to his disputations, enthusiasms and support.

TIM ALBERT
Leatherhead
February 2000

Preface to the first edition

This book stems from my conviction that writing a scientific paper is not as hard as many people are led to believe. Most books on the subject, while scholarly and informative, take the task very seriously, thereby leaving readers with the impression that they are in for a hard time.

This book takes a different approach: it aims to raise standards not by printing rules but by encouraging more people to have a go. This is not to say that knowledge and scholarship are not important; they are. But we need to supplement them with enthusiasm, a quality that often seems hard to find when it comes to writing articles. I hope that, when you come to the end, this book will have inspired you to have written.

The quotations at the start of nine chapters originate from written coursework for a workshop on the writing process given to members of the European Medical Writers Association in 1995 and 1996. The quotation at the head of Chapter 2 is a verbal comment from a participant at the end of a Postgraduate course in Holland entitled *How to write a scientific paper*.

I would like to thank those who have helped me in various ways to write this book. Most important, perhaps, are all those students I have taught over the past five years and who have inspired me to re-evaluate my existing skills and learn new ones. Those who taught with me accelerated this process, and I am therefore grateful to Gordon Macpherson, Bill Whimster, Harvey Marcovitch, Norma Pearce and Jane Dawson.

I would also like to thank those who have read and commented on versions of this book, including those mentioned above and also Geert-Jan van Daal, Jane Donovan, Neville Goodman, Richard Horton, Louis Hue and Pete Moore. I would also like to express my thanks to Richard Smith for agreeing to write the Foreword. Last but not least, I would like to thank my wife Barbara for putting up with my unsocial behaviour during the writing of this book.

Tim Albert
Leatherhead
August 1996

Introduction
Is it still worth learning how to write scientific papers?

In the four short years since this book was published, the world of scientific publishing has started to come to terms with the most important development since the birth of the printing press. The question I faced, when deciding whether to produce a second edition, was whether the craft of writing a scientific paper was still worth writing about – or whether churning out yet another book on the topic would turn out to have been as useful as urging Noah's offspring to forget the fancy boat-building and concentrate on the ploughshares.

The changes began with the development of the personal computer, the impact of which was already being felt three years ago. Less than a generation ago, we visited libraries to research the literature, leafing through leather-bound editions and taking notes on paper. We used the new calculators to add up columns of numbers and drew figures by hand. We took a pen or pencil to write the first draft, working through several sets before we came to the one that satisfied us.

Now we can search the databases from our homes, downloading articles that interest us and assembling them into lists of references, with style adjusted for our target journal. When we feed in raw data, the computer does the calculations and produces a range of charts and graphs within seconds. We write straight onto the computer, which tells us when we make errors of grammar or spelling, and enables us to make immediate corrections.

These are all basically labour-saving devices, whose main implication is to have made writing a little less unpleasant. The real shock waves are coming from the development of the world wide web. This has thrown down a challenge to the traditional view of the scientific paper, which until now has had two main disadvantages. First, costs rose in direct relation to the amount of material being distributed and to the number of people it was being distributed to. Second, once the paper was printed, it was frozen in time and stopped developing. The challenge set by electronic publishing is that, with its huge capacity to add information and readers at no additional cost, many of the current structures are no longer needed.

Publishers, therefore, face a range of key questions. Who will be given access to these new electronic journals? How will they be funded? Who will guarantee quality? Will publishers actually have a role, or will individuals and groups start to publish their own research?

Whatever happens, there will be massive changes, though the time scale is going to be slightly longer than the five years predicted by a group of writers in 1997.[1] New players are emerging, such as fully electronic journals. Traditional paper-based journals are running into trouble, as libraries cut down on the journals they subscribe to and as the more prestigious journals start to publish shorter versions on paper while posting longer versions on their web site, thereby giving them room to accept more papers.

Far from harming writers, this is likely to benefit them by simplifying the present system. Authors will have fewer pub-lications to choose from – and argue over with co-authors. Journals, freed from the restrictions of space, will be able to publish on the basis of quality alone, and not availability of pages. Selection will become less unfair.

Another change that will help writers is likely to be an element of greater standardisation. As electronic links grow, there is likely to be greater pressure for standardising titles. These could move towards the *BMJ* style (topic and methods linked by a colon) or towards the current fashion in US journals to have declarative titles (with a verb). The cornerstone of the scientific paper – the IMRAD structure – may also become more standardised, ending up as little more than a list. This has happened already with the structured abstract and seems to be spreading with proposals for a structured discussion.[2] A new standardised language, based on US usage, is also likely to emerge, partly because of demand from consumers, and partly because our (US-made) software will steer us in this direction anyway. (Already we are beginning to capitalise the first word in titles, to use a capital letter after a colon, and to favour '-ize' rather than '-ise'.)

At the same time authors will have greater opportunities to be creative. In theory there will be no limitation on the amount of text they submit (perhaps not an undisputed benefit!). They will be able to set up imaginative links that will send inquirers to the original data, to earlier or related studies, or even to a picture of the clinic where the work was done. Refinements can be added, such as better graphics, more colour and moving images. Authors will be able to write in different styles for different structures, according to the preferences of whoever happens to be reading.

This leads to the most welcome implication of all. With all the turgid information stored and validated in standardised form on the databases, web sites and paper-based journals will be able to revert to the original role of journals – not to validate science but to communicate its exciting advances. Already some are becoming much more accessible, bringing in mainstream journalism techniques such as pictorial covers with beckoning cover-lines, dynamic contents pages with cross-references to later articles, photographs and cartoons, and even (in some still fairly isolated cases) a move back to a language that is not jargon-ridden, but accessible to all.

All this, of course, will have enormous implications for authors. Within the time needed for a new edition to have sold out, our notion of a 'good paper' will have changed and therefore many of the elements included in this book will have become redundant. This could be depressing for all of us – author, publisher and you, dear reader – were it not for the fact that this book tries to go further than equipping people to meet the current view of a 'good paper'. Its somewhat broader view is based on some key lessons. Write only if you have to. If you do have to write, think carefully about your message. Analyse carefully what you are being asked to write and meet those 'market requirements'. Finally, don't allow yourself to be discouraged by those who pretend that a scientific paper is somehow different from, or harder than, any other type of writing.

I suspect that these skills will remain useful as long as there is a need to communicate in writing, whatever the means of delivery.

References

1   Bero L and Dalamothe T *et al.* (1997) The electronic future. *BMJ.* **315**: 1692–6.

2   Docherty M and Smith R (1998) The case for structuring the discussion of scientific papers. *BMJ.* **381**: 1224–5.

1

Know the game

'Writing is a highly individual and intensely personal process and I doubt that there are any general rules which would apply to everyone.'

The process of writing

The purpose of this book is to enable you to write, and to have published, a scientific paper or article in a peer-reviewed journal – in other words to have your name on the established databases. It is not a book about how to 'do science', but a book on how to translate the science you do into publishable papers.

The driving force has come from what I have seen over the past 10 years, while giving several hundred courses on effective writing to doctors and other scientists. What struck me was that:

1 many of them felt that they would be failures unless they became published authors
2 few of them had actually been given practical advice on how to do this.

Conspiracy theorists would have a field day. They would argue that those who have discovered the secret of publication are, for obvious reasons, unwilling to pass it on to younger rivals. That is clearly untrue. There is no shortage of senior scientists willing to devote much time to helping junior colleagues, and there are dozens of worthy books explaining in great detail the criteria for acceptable scientific articles.

Yet somehow all this energy achieves little, and many people who want to write remain confused and unable to start. To some extent this is a particular characteristic of science writing, which has become highly specialised and removed from other types of writing. Many 'experts' discuss in great detail exactly what conditions a 'good' article should fulfil, but few promote, or even seem aware of, some of the useful techniques of how to get started and write it.

However, there is a wealth of information on the *process* of writing, which is readily accessible to those who go outside the world of science into the world of professional communicators. That is the gap this book tries to fill, by treating writing tasks, quite simply, as writing tasks, and by applying the (mainstream) techniques and tricks of the professional writer to the (specialist) world of scientific writing. This may be considered radical, and some of the ideas may give offence. But I believe strongly that there are basic principles of effective writing that can be applied to all types of writing. It can work. As one participant once wrote to me: 'Before your course I'd had an article rejected by the *BMJ*. After the course I rewrote it and it was accepted by *The Lancet*'.

This book divides the process of writing into ten easy steps. Some of the main problems that this book addresses, and the chapters where their resolution may be found, are given in Figure 1.1. What I hope shines through is that, despite the inevitable episodes of pain (such as these opening seven paragraphs which took at least 20 drafts), writing should be fun. It should also be rewarding and even liberating. This is not an impossible dream: it depends more than anything else on the writer's frame of mind, and therefore is quite easy to fix.

If that sounds like one of those motivational books, so be it. That is precisely what I hope this book will be.

Figure 1.1: Common problems faced by writers

I don't have enough time to write	see Chapters 2,3
I haven't got any good ideas	see Chapter 3
I don't know how to get started	see Chapter 3
I write too much	see Chapters 3, 4
I find it difficult to stop researching	see Chapter 4
I find it difficult to structure my writing	see Chapter 5
I find writing slow and painful	see Chapter 6
I make mistakes of spelling and/or grammar	see Chapter 7
I don't know when to write the title and abstract	see Chapter 8
Other people keep changing what I write	see Chapter 9
I don't know whom to send my article to	see Chapter 10
I don't know if I've written a good article	see Chapter 10

The scientific article as truth

There are many different types of scientific writing (Figure 1.2), but this book focuses on how to write an original scientific article or paper (the terms seem interchangeable). I have chosen to focus on them because they have become the staple currency of scientific writing. They have also adopted a particular format, and on the face of it seem least likely to share common ground with other types of writing. In fact I believe the reverse is true: there are principles of effective writing that you can use to master scientific articles, and that you can also use for all other types of writing, including reports, letters, memos, grant submissions and patient information.

Scientific articles have a long history. The first reviewed paper is generally considered to date from the middle 17th century, and a series of developments since (Figure 1.3) have led to a process that is today complex, sophisticated and international. The basic form of a scientific article consists of a 2000–3000 word report that normally addresses a single research question. It uses a standard structure of introduction, methods, results and discussion (the IMRAD structure, of

***

Figure 1.2: Different types of scientific writing

Original article	A new piece of knowledge we lay claim to (2000–3000 words, sometimes more)
Case report	A single event that could lead to a new piece of knowledge we could lay claim to (600 words)
Review article	Knowledge others have laid claim to (2000 words)
Editorial	What I think of the knowledge that others have laid claim to (800 words)
Book review	What I think of a piece of knowledge that someone else is claiming (400 words)
Letters	What I think of the knowledge claims in your journals (400 words)

Distinguish from . . .

Examination essay	What I can put down on paper, within a given time limit, about the various claims of knowledge from other people

***

Figure 1.3: Some key dates in the evolution of scientific publishing[1]

1665	First scientific journals in France and the UK
1820s	First specialist journals
1870s	References began to be collected at the end of articles
1920s	First summaries appeared at the end of articles
1930s	First papers on the use of statistics
1950s	Widespread acceptance of the IMRAD format
1960s	Summaries at the end became abstracts at the beginning
1970s	Databases introduced
1980s	First international conference on peer review
1990s	Introduction of electronic journals

which much more later), plus other specific items, such as title, abstract, key words and list of references. These articles are written in a particularly stylised form of English.

One or several authors submit an article to the editor of a journal. The editors have knowledge and integrity, according to the conventional view, and act as gatekeepers, selecting the 'good' and rejecting the 'bad'. They are assisted by a complex system of peer review, under which a few people working in the same field are invited to give their opinion.

The criteria on which papers are accepted are generally considered to include the following:

- original: is the work new?
- significant: does it represent an important advance?
- first disclosure: has it appeared in print elsewhere?
- reproducible: can the work be repeated?

Each week thousands of these papers appear, in publications ranging from international general journals, sometimes run by multi-national publishing groups, to small specialist journals published by a group of doctors in one country and who share a common professional interest. Many of these papers are now available in abstract form on international databases, thus ensuring that, within a short period of completing the work, the findings are available throughout the world. Many of the journals are now publishing electronically.

The system is impressive. Week by week our knowledge grows as original articles – the basic building blocks of science – are approved, published and disseminated. It's a powerful thought and a comforting view.

The truth about scientific articles

It also happens to be a naive and unduly rosy view. Dr Stephen Lock, former editor of the *British Medical Journal*, has written:

'The journals are serving the community poorly. Many articles are neither read nor cited; indeed many articles are poor. In general, medical journals seem to be of little practical help to clinicians facing problems at the bedside . . . Scientific articles have been hijacked away from their primary role of communicating scientific discovery to one of demonstrating academic activity. No more are grant-giving bodies basing awards on the quality of scientific research; the research has switched to quantity'[1] (see Bookchoice p. 9).

The performance of journals does not always live up to the glowing picture painted of them. One major problem is that the peer-review system, for all its intricacies, does not guarantee that the bad will be weeded out or even that the good will be published in the most appropriate journal. There has been a small but steady stream of cases where an author copied data from a previously published article (plagiarism), published the same article twice (duplicate publication), or simply invented data (fraud). A notorious example in the UK concerned a short report on the successful transplantation of an ectopic pregnancy into the womb. It later emerged that the whole thing was an invention. But it had passed through the system, and was only discovered when an insider 'blew the whistle'.[2]

Nor do all the efforts of reviewing guarantee that papers will be good, as opposed to mediocre. The comments of others can be invaluable, but they can also have the effect of promoting conservatism and disparaging innovation. There is a danger that, by the time articles are passed for publication, they carry the stamp of agreement by committee and have lost any spark of individuality. Most serious of all is the charge that the reviewers may provide unwitting bias on the one hand, and on the other downright chicanery (as one research team tries to discredit the results of a rival or use the information in a refereed paper to further its own research).

All this makes life extremely difficult as far as writers are concerned. Publication is not just a matter of adding to intellectual debate and seeing your name in print. Nowadays it is (curiously and for no apparent reason other than it is easily measurable) one of the main factors taken into account when assessing the worth of individuals and research groups.

Unfortunately, this can be extremely unfair, as illustrated by a story told by a young researcher on a course. He had written a paper which had been accepted for publication by a reputable journal. He scanned the journal for months – in vain. Eventually he telephoned the editorial staff. He was told that the article had been mislaid but, now that it had been found, it could not be published because the editor felt that the figures were now out of date. The author was heartbroken. In his eyes, he had fulfilled the criteria, but did not receive the kudos, or the points for his CV. At the same time the editor was well within his rights. If he felt that the readers would not be interested, then it would have been wrong to have published it.

At heart is the harsh reality that our main method of validating science is ultimately based on a commercial system. Editors have many roles and have to reconcile many pressures (Figure 1.4). But one of their main tasks is to ensure that the publication continues to exist. For this, articles must be read and cited. If this no longer happens, then the journal will have

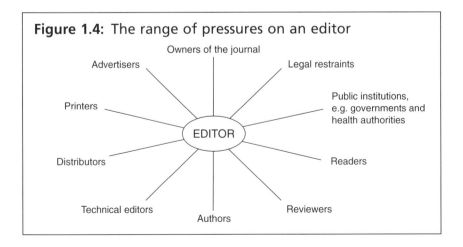

Figure 1.4: The range of pressures on an editor

Owners of the journal

Advertisers

Legal restraints

Printers

Public institutions, e.g. governments and health authorities

EDITOR

Distributors

Readers

Technical editors

Reviewers

Authors

to close. As Lawrence K Altman, the medical correspondent of the *New York Times*, has reminded us: 'Scientific journals represent scholarship. But they are also an industry. Medical and surgical journals in North America collect more than $3 billion in advertising revenue each year'.[3]

The traditional idea – that a 'good paper' will automatically receive the recognition it deserves – is clearly unrealistic. But where does this leave the aspiring writer?

Marketing – a comforting but vulgar approach

The way out of this mess is to stop thinking of scientific papers as a way of assessing individual worth, and more as part of a commercial publishing system. Journals need good articles and every editor's ultimate nightmare is that there will not be enough copy to fill the journal. As a potential supplier, you have a marvellous opportunity: if you can provide the right product for the right market, you will achieve your sale – and be published.

This means redefining yourself as a supplier and your purpose as making a sale. The end product is not necessarily what colleagues think is a 'good paper' but one that has been published in the journal of your choice. There are several advantages to this approach. You have a clear way in which to measure your success. If (or rather when) failure comes along and a paper is rejected, you can take comfort from the fact that this does not make you an incompetent doctor and a failed human being. Like many other producers, you will have made a faulty marketing decision. You will also, of course, have learnt a valuable lesson for next time.

Some find this vulgar and argue that it is devaluing science to talk about scientific papers in overtly commercial terms. It reflects reality. I am not encouraging you to write rubbish or to invent data; though I am encouraging you to see writing as a craft that can be learnt, not as a gift from the gods. Stripping away some of the mythology surrounding scientific papers and the world of journals should encourage more and more writers to have a go. And this in turn should raise standards.

Implications for the reader of this book

What this means for you, as an intending writer, is that you should stop being intimidated by those who appear to be more successful at writing than you. Take them less seriously; treat the writing business as a game. The rules are simple: when you have written a paper that has been published in your journal of first choice, you are the winner.

Before proceeding to Chapter 2 you should:
- understand that you can win the publications game by becoming a published author. Do not let others discourage you.

BOOKCHOICE: The role of medical journals

Lock S (ed) (1991) *The Future of Medical Journals*. BMJ Publications, London.

In 1991 the *British Medical Journal* organised a prestigious conference to mark its 150th anniversary. Those invited to present papers at a Kent castle were the great and the good of medical journals on both sides of the Atlantic. Although it is nearly 10 years since the book of the proceedings was published, it remains one of the best and most provocative books on a broad range of medical publishing issues.

Stephen Lock, then the outgoing editor of the *BMJ*, sets the scene with a forthright introduction on the shortcomings of present journals. The book also deals with most of the major issues facing scientific publishing. How can we judge the effectiveness of journals? What is their future, particularly in view of the arrival of electronic publishing? What is the role of meta-analysis? What should be the relationship between clinical practice and research? What should we do about the 'technical, anaemic and tribalistic' language which authors assume is expected? All these are important questions for those running the academic publication industry.

The book ends on a positive note with a paper from Richard Smith, Dr Lock's successor as editor of the *BMJ*: 'I believe that the future for general medical journals – particularly those published in English – is bright. They will undoubtedly change, but they will not disappear. Electronic forms of publishing will become increasingly important after a hesitant start, but general journals will continue to exist in hard copy – not least because that is the comfortable way to read, particularly in the bath, but also because of the importance of serendipity in reading and learning. Indeed, the buffeting and transforming of the medical profession over the next few decades will return general medical journals to their central function of gluing the profession together'. His predictions seem, so far, to be coming true.

2

Know yourself

'I think I'd rather go fishing.'

Do you really want to write?

The most important component of a scientific paper is not the data. It is you.

If you seriously wish to become a published author, you will have to make certain changes in your life. You will face added hours of solitary work and many frustrations. You will have to call on reserves of tact, optimism and determination. At one stage you could even discover that you are creating a monster that is threatening to take over parts of your life (and the lives of your loved ones).

Not surprisingly, many people drop out along the way. They end up with half-finished manuscripts, or a head-full of promising ideas that go around and around – but never forward. They may well be those who are loudest in telling you exactly how you should be writing. They may appear contemptuous of anything anyone else has written, but in reality this serves to disguise the fact that they wish that they had got there first.

What marks out a writer from the rest of the world is simple: the writer has found time to start – and finish – the writing task. The key factor is not so much knowledge or skills but time management. Successful authors are those who have managed their resources more effectively.

As a starting point, you must be absolutely clear *why* you want to be published in the first place. This is one of those deceptively simple questions that, once you have dared to pose it, brings out all kinds of motives that might have been better unroused.

The most common motive is one that people tend to be embarrassed about: publication is necessary to advance your career. There is no need to be ashamed. This is a fact of contemporary life, and if you don't compete you will lose out. Whether you approve of it or not is irrelevant.

Some writers say that their motive is to share with others what they have discovered. Others take a self-exploratory view: writing a paper is a test of self-worth. Or, as with climbing mountains, they do it simply because it is there. Then there are the missionaries, who take the position that they have a duty to write because everyone else is publishing rubbish.

Whichever motives you choose to admit to in public, in private you must be completely honest with yourself. Unless you know why you want to publish, how can you gauge whether you are progressing towards your goals? I fondly remember one course participant, who said after the second day that he had greatly enjoyed himself and learnt a great deal about the mechanics of writing a paper. But, he continued, he had a busy and successful practice and a growing family, and he had now come to the conclusion that he would make a better use of his time by going fishing instead.

He was in control.

Goals – and can you achieve them?

Once you know why you feel you should be writing, you can start setting some realistic writing goals. If you want to be a professor before the age of 38, for instance, then you may decide that you need to have published three papers in prestigious journals within the next year. If you wish to write one paper for your CV then a different set of actions would be in order (Figure 2.1).

Make sure that you are in a position to do what you need to do. You have a problem, for instance, if you need to publish an original paper and the only material you come across is suitable for case reports. You may have to set up your own research, or find a new job where you can spend more time on research. But modern life is not always as straightforward as that, and you may not be able to take such drastic action. Furthermore, you may be part of a larger team, and have little influence on what you can write. The important thing is that you keep a sense of reality: do not write yourself off as an incompetent writer when in fact, through no fault of your own, you have nothing suitable to write about.

Making time

How are you going to find time? Writing will always use more of this scarce commodity than you expect. We all share the set quota of 24 hours a day; what distinguishes us from each other is how we decide to fill these hours. This will inevitably mean that something must go.

You may find it less painful if you can keep writing tasks to a set time each week. This will help you to get into a routine. Many successful writers manage to do without some of their sleep, and get up, say, at five in the morning. You might find

Figure 2.1: Setting your writing goals

Version A: What is your writing goal?
Three papers in prestigious journals within the next 12 months so that I can become a professor before the age of 38.

What can you provide?
Study A provisionally accepted; study B just finishing final draft; study C needs final data.

How will you find time to write?
Fifteen minutes every evening before going to bed, and two hours on Sunday morning.

What are your writing objectives for the next six months?
1 Amend article A, provisionally accepted by *The Lancet*, and send off within one week
2 Write letter to editor for article B
3 Send article B, plus letter to editor, to co-authors for final approval within two weeks
4 Set the brief on article C within four weeks
5 Review within six weeks.

Version B: What is your writing goal?
Bolster my CV with one article in a reasonable journal.

What can you provide?
One case history. Possible major study with two other centres.

How will you find time to write?
Two weeks between jobs. Then evenings.

What are your writing objectives for the next six months?
1 Decide whether to do the case history or the major study
2 Make appointment with head of department to seek advice
3 Buy word processor
4 Finish this book
5 Review in three months.

this too drastic, but you could go without a favourite television programme, or put aside a couple of hours a week on a Sunday evening. Don't feel you have to allocate huge chunks of time. Fifteen minutes a day, six days a week will help you to make steady progress; it should also help you to maintain your enthusiasm.

Some people say they will find time when they need to. This is not a recommended option, mainly because there is an easier way.

Setting objectives

Now you know what you need to write, and how you will find the necessary time, all that remains is to spend a little time deciding what you have to do to get there. These tasks will be your objectives.

Do not confuse objectives with vague ambitions. Most people, when asked to suggest their writing objectives, come up with enormous tasks such as:

- write three papers within six months
- finish my PhD before the holidays
- get something (anything!) published within two years.

Make your objectives attainable. They could be simple tasks, like reading the *Instructions to authors* from a target journal, or reading a book (or perhaps just finishing this one), or drawing up some tables of your data. These are all tasks that you will need to complete, and you will find life much more satisfying if you make steady progress – and can acknowledge that fact.

Put a realistic time limit on each objective, and a time limit, such as six months or a year, on the whole series. Make time to review these regularly. After a few months you will start to realise that you are beginning to achieve what you set out to achieve. After a year you could well be surprised by how far you have come.

> Before proceeding to Chapter 3 you should:
> - be absolutely clear why you want to write, how you can achieve this goal, and when you will achieve it. Write it down.

3

First set yourself a brief

'Step one: think about what to write on the tram on the way to work.'

When to stop researching and start writing

One of the main reasons why writing fails is that the reader cannot find in it a clear message. This is usually because the writer has failed to put one in, probably because he or she started to write too early. Good writing is rooted in good thought, and this preparatory stage, which involves taking time to think about what you are writing, is vital. It is often neglected.

If you have got this far you presumably have some idea of what you wish to write. You may only have a hypothesis or a protocol; on the other hand you may well have your kitchen table groaning with data. Resist the temptation to go straight to the word processor and do not believe those who say you should start putting your ideas on paper as soon as possible. Do a literature search and try sketching in some of the introduction, they might say, or write down what you have done so far for the methods. Perhaps you can jot down some ideas on the harder bits, like the discussion, and before you know where you are, you've nearly finished . . .

This is not a sensible way to proceed. With no clear vision, you will become obsessed with detail. You will fiddle with figures, chase up obscure references and have long disputes with your colleagues over everything from typography to grammar. At best this will delay and demoralise; at worst it will destroy the whole project.

You wouldn't dream of behaving in this way when you drive a car. You don't jump in and start driving. You work out where your destination is and the best route for getting there. All sensible business people take care to do comprehensive planning and market research before launching a new product, yet all over the world doctors and researchers invest time and egos in writing papers that – were they to think them through properly from the start – they would realise have major flaws and are unlikely ever to be published.

Set aside some time to think and make this part of the process. I call this stage *setting the brief* (a term that comes from the jargon of journalism). Some people do this informally, or even subconsciously, but I recommend that it becomes a major ritual, to be undertaken at the start of any major writing project. Take as much time as you need – and make sure that you commit your decisions to paper. Once you have completed it, you will be through the worst and you will have made decisions in five key areas:

1 the message
2 the market
3 the length
4 the deadline
5 the co-authors.

This process of setting the brief marks the time when the research ends and the writing starts. You will, of course, revisit your data, but the relationship between research and writing has subtly changed. From now on the piece of writing becomes the master, and the data its servant. This is the best way of ensuring that, at the end of the process, you will have written something that others will clearly understand.

Only one message per article

Scientific papers are expected to communicate findings to other people. To do this successfully, you need to do more than throw a number of facts on to a piece of paper. You need to organise or structure them, so that the relationship between the various items of information becomes clear. If you organise successfully, there will be a common theme, which the reader will be able to pull out as a single thought. This is your message.

The problem with any piece of research, and any piece of writing, is that the number of potential messages is vast. Many people try to skirt round the challenge of working out which is the most important, or they try to fit them all in anyway. That is why so much writing fails: the reader is unable to come away with a clear message. Readers usually blame themselves for not being clever enough to understand, but almost always the fault lies with the writer.

Do not expect a clear message to emerge as you write. This is like putting a pile of bricks together and expecting a house to arise. There is only one way of ensuring that your writing is focused on one simple message, and that is by defining this message carefully before you start. To keep it as clear as possible, you should express it as one sentence of 10–14 words, with a verb.

Imagine, for example, that you have spent the past five years conducting a trial to see whether Obecalp is an effective treatment for post-lunchtime amnesia in doctors. You may think the results are so momentous that you couldn't possibly confine them to one sentence. But try, and you will immediately, and with little difficulty, come up with a number of alternatives.

1 Obecalp is an effective treatment for post-lunchtime amnesia.
2 Obecalp is an effective treatment for post-lunchtime amnesia in doctors if given within 48 hours of onset.
3 This latest piece of research adds to the evidence that Obecalp may be an effective treatment.

All could be perfectly good messages for a piece of writing. All are plausible and, presumably, supported by the evidence. The information will, broadly speaking, be the same for each. But the exact form your writing takes will vary tremendously, depending on which message you have chosen to convey.

Making this decision is not an easy task. It should not be done in a darkened room facing a word processor or blank piece of paper. It should be done in what Henriette Anne Klauser calls 'rumination time',[4] on the move – travelling to work or going for a walk or riding a bicycle. It needs a clear(ish) head, a moderate amount of time, a pencil and a scrap of paper (used envelopes are particularly suitable) on which you will write down your thoughts. Feel free to talk your ideas through with other people – but remember that you are the one who is going to do the writing, and you are the one who has to decide on the message. (See also Bookchoice, p. 58.)

Use the language of the public house or coffee house rather than the private journal. Far from limiting thought, this should clarify it. Which version is more specific? 'Obecalp is now clearly indicated as the treatment of choice for post-lunchtime amnesia', or one of the following?

1 Doctors should immediately prescribe Obecalp to all those suffering from post-lunchtime amnesia.

2   Researchers need to test Obecalp on more people before we can decide whether we should use it.
3   Obecalp cured three of the four rats with post-lunchtime amnesia.

Do not confuse the message with a title. We shall return to titles in Chapter 8, but at this stage the point to stress is that writing a title now could positively hinder your progress over the next few weeks. As shown in Figure 3.1, a message will give you the direction you are going to take; a title will normally indicate only which broad area you are to cover. Similarly, at this stage we do not want a question; we want the answer.

Choosing the market

Once you have decided on your message, ask: in which journal do you intend to have it published? This is another difficult question, and again many authors delay their decision until after they have written. Perhaps they hope that the solution will emerge as they move along the writing process, or that the finished project will somehow be so good that every editor will be fighting to take it.

Nevertheless, there are resounding arguments for matching message to market at this early stage. You can make an informed decision, before you start committing time and energy, as to whether the publication you are considering is likely to publish an article of the type you are about to write. It is better to do this now than it is to discover, too late, that you have been writing an article that no one is likely to publish. Another advantage is that, once you have decided on the target journal, you will have published evidence that will guide you as you go through the writing process, and will help you later as you come to discuss your work with your colleagues. Find a

---

Figure 3.1: Titles versus messages

On the left are titles as used in the *BMJ* (July 31, 1999). On the right are the headlines on the summaries of these papers which appeared as short news items in the front of the journal. Note that the titles give the subject, but the headlines, all of which have verbs, give messages. When writing an article, the message will be a defining, and more useful, starting point than a title.

Title	Message
Randomised controlled trial of exercise for low back pain: clinical outcomes, costs, and preferences	Community exercise classes help people with back pain
Long term vascular complications of *Coxiella burnetii* infection in Switzerland: cohort study	*Coxiella burnetii* infection may be linked to cardiovascular disease
Prospective risk of unexplained stillbirth in singleton pregnancies at term: population based analysis	Unexpected late stillbirths are more common than sudden infant deaths
Near patient testing for respiratory syncytial virus in paediatric accident and emergency: prospective pilot study	Near patient test for respiratory syncytial virus identifies positive cases
Effect of mass media campaign to reduce socioeconomic differences in women's awareness and behaviour concerning use of folic acid: cross-sectional study.	Mass media campaign on folic acid did not alter socioeconomic differences

---

copy of the *Instructions to authors* (Figure 3.2); this should be your constant companion over the weeks to come.

All this is obvious. In practice the problem is: how do you choose the target journal in the first place? There is no easy answer. The message you wish to put across will be a useful starting point and should narrow the field considerably.

Figure 3.2: Instructions to authors

All journals publish *Instructions to authors*, in which they lay down their requirements and their philosophy. They are vital pieces of information, and prospective authors must study them closely and often, both while choosing a target journal and subsequently working on the manuscript.

On one level they give precise instructions in important areas such as how to present the manuscript, how many copies to provide, where to send it and so on. They also deal with some of the issues that come with publication, such as copyright assignment and whether offprints are supplied. On a more subtle level, they will give you a valuable flavour of the journal's personality and, presumably, that of the editor(s). Compare, for instance, these two contrasting extracts:

1 'The ARCHIVES [of dermatology] desires to publish clinical and laboratory studies that enhance the understanding of skin and its diseases. In addition to these STUDIES, case reports that substantially add to our knowledge in a meaningful fashion will be published as OBSERVATIONS.
   The CIRCULATION of the ARCHIVES is among the highest of any dermatological publication in the world – currently 14 000. The journal is received by virtually all requesting US physicians – including academicians and second- and third-year residents – who practise dermatology as their primary specialty as self-designated in the AMA Physician Masterfile.'

2 '*The British Journal of Dermatology* publishes original articles on all aspects of the biology and pathology of the skin. Originally the journal, founded in 1888, was devoted almost exclusively to the interests of the dermatologist in clinical practise. However, the rapid development, since the 1950s, of research on the physiology and experimental pathology of the skin has been reflected in the contents of the Journal, which now provides a vehicle for the publication of both experimental and clinical ethical research and serves equally the laboratory worker and the clinician.'

Another consideration is what you want to get out of publication. (Chapter 2 should have helped you with this.) If you want fame across the profession, then aim for a general journal, such as *Nature*, *The Lancet*, *BMJ* or *New England Journal of Medicine*. If you seek promotion, then go for those with the highest impact factors (Figure 3.3). If you want to influence a small group of doctors only, then choose a specialist journal.

You may wish to produce a shortlist of four or five journals. If you still find it difficult to choose, run a literature search.

Figure 3.3: Citation reports and impact factors

Eugene Garfield's grand idea was that he could produce league tables of journals by counting the number of times each paper published in each journal was subsequently cited by other authors. This led to the Institute for Scientific Information and the annual *Journal Citation Reports*.[5] 'By tabulating and aggregating citations', says the Institute, 'the *Journal Citation Reports* offers a unique perspective for journal evaluation and comparison'.

The main measures are:

- journal size: calculated by the number of articles
- most frequently used: the number of times they are cited
- 'hottest journals': number of times a journal's current articles are cited in the year in which they are published
- impact factor: number of current citations to articles published in previous two years.

Like all league tables, these attract arguments for and against. But, as the Institute points out, they do help authors 'to choose where to publish, discover new and foreign publications in their specialty, and select a "shortlist" of journals to be scanned regularly for current awareness'.

a The ten most cited scientific journals

Rank	Journal	Citations
1	*J Biol Chem*	322 529
2	*Proc Natl Acad Sci USA*	290 121
3	*Nature*	288 026
4	*Science*	250 327
5	*J Am Chem Soc*	179 036
6	*Cell*	159 685
7	*Phys Rev B*	146 573
8	*Phys Rev Lett*	134 476
9	*N Engl J Med*	129 928
10	*J Chem Phys*	115 941

Figure 3.3 (*continued*)

b The ten highest-impact scientific journals

Rank	Journal	Impact factor
1	*Ann Rev Immunol*	42.9
2	*Nat Genet*	40.4
3	*Annu Rev Biochem*	39.0
4	*Cell*	38.7
5	*Nature*	28.8
6	*N Engl J Med*	28.7
7	*Nat Med*	27.9
8	*Science*	24.4
9	*Physiol Rev*	23.7
10	*Ann Rev Neurosci*	23.0

c The ten highest-impact general medical journals

Rank	Journal	Impact factor
1	*N Engl J Med*	28.7
2	*Lancet*	11.8
3	*Ann Intern Med*	10.9
4	*JAMA*	9.6
5	*Annu Rev Med*	5.9
6	*Arch Intern Med*	5.4
7	*BMJ*	5.3
8	*Am J Med*	4.4
9	*J Invest Med*	3.8
10	*Medicine*	3.7

How much has each of them published about your subject in the past few years? You will find that journals, like their editors, show patterns of interest – preferences for dealing with certain topics and shunning others. This piece of market research should help you to make an informed decision, but if you still find it hard to decide, choose a journal you read and enjoy because, as a regular reader, you will be comfortable with its style and approach.

Do not be shy of ambition. If you want (or need) to be published in a top journal, study that journal closely. Look at the articles in your specialty it has run recently. Can you provide, and support, a message of comparable quality? If so, there is no reason why you should not be able to become published, irrespective of your (current) place in the hierarchy.

The length

How long should your article be? The answer now becomes quite simple. It is what your target journal requires. You should find this covered in the *Instructions to authors*; but you would do well to take some articles and count the paragraphs; these are a more manageable unit than words alone. The principle is that length is determined not by how much you wish to write, but by what the market will bear.

You will doubtless feel you need more space to do yourself justice; everyone does. Remember the story (probably apocryphal, because I hear it attributed to different writers depending on which country I'm in) about the literary figure who wrote: 'I apologise for such a long letter; I didn't have time to write a short one'. It conveys an important truth: all writing can be shortened. It will make life harder for you, but easier for your reader.

Deadlines

Having a plan of what to write, and for whom, won't give you the necessary momentum unless you put a deadline on it. The previous chapter stressed the importance of this.

But you should do more than set a deadline; set several. Writing and submitting a scientific article is a huge task, and unless you approach it with cunning, the nearer you get to it the further away it will seem to move. Break this large task down into smaller ones: the first of which could be to set yourself a deadline for deciding on your message. Give yourself, say, five days.

Be honest with yourself. I have seen some wonderful excuses over the past five years, from 'absence of our secretary', 'unplanned trip to the United States', 'illness of our figure drawer' to 'my husband left me and took the laser printer'. By all means use such excuses to deal with outsiders, but under no account should you start fooling yourself.

Co-authors

Writing is a personal activity. Someone has to do the solitary tasks like thinking, planning, writing, rewriting, and arbitrating between opposing views. If you are the person who is doing all this, then you have a sound moral case to be the first author. As such, you are in effect the team leader, and the responsibility of managing the project is yours.

Resist the notion of writing in committee. Committees are not suitable because the emphasis inevitably switches from pleasing the target reader to pleasing those sitting round the table. You will need contributions from other members of the team, but it will be your responsibility to solicit them individually, make decisions about them, and generally reconcile opposing views.

Whom should you name as your co-authors? Here there is not only potential conflict between you and your colleagues, but between you and your future editor. Editors over the years have been influenced by clear cases of abuse or 'ghost authorship', when people who had no right to share the credit have insisted that their names be included. They now take a tough line and say that authorship should be based only on 'substantial contributions' (Figure 3.4). This cuts little ice with those who see clearly that getting their name on a paper will increase considerably their chances of progressing in their

Figure 3.4: The editor's view of authorship

According to the Vancouver Group of editors: 'All persons designated as authors should qualify for authorship. Each author should have participated sufficiently in the work to take public responsibility for the content.

Authorship credit should be based only on substantial contributions to:

a conception and design, or analysis and interpretation of data, and on

b drafting the article or revising it critically for important intellectual content, and on

c final approval of the version to be published.

Conditions a, b and c must all be met. Participation solely in the acquisition of funding or the collection of data does not justify authorship. General supervision of the research group is not sufficient for authorship. Any part of an article critical to its main conclusions must be the responsibility of at least one author. Editors may ask authors to describe what each contributed; this information may be published.'

For further information on the Vancouver Group, see page 33.

careers. This is really a political question, not a writing one. First authors have to compromise, particularly if those who wish to be associated as co-authors are higher up the hierarchy. What you must guard against is having so many co-authors that your paper starts to look ridiculous, such as 12 authors reporting tests on three dogs. There comes a point where it could jeopardise your chances of publication.

One way of reducing the strain is to negotiate on all aspects of the question of authorship before you start the writing. Work out as far as possible who will be your co-authors, and what the role of each of them will be. This should eliminate some of the worst excesses. It should also ease the strain in the latter stages of the writing process, when many hours can be wasted because the co-authors – without realising it – are actually trying to write different papers with different

Figure 3.5: Setting the brief

Example A

Message: A multi-national trial of 2373 post-lunchtime amnesia sufferers has shown that Obecalp is more effective than the established treatment.

Market: *The Lancet*

Length: 2500 words

Deadline: First draft by July 13

Co-authors: All those involved in the seven centres.

Example B

Message: 36 out of 40 patients with chronic post-lunchtime amnesia went into immediate remission after a diet of dandelion leaves and frankfurters.

Market: *Journal of the Society of Postprandial Pathologists*

Length: 4000 words

Deadline: First draft by tomorrow week

Co-authors: The medical student who first spotted it and the consultant you report to.

messages. Before you go any further, send them in writing a copy of the message you propose, and ask if they agree.

Also make sure at this stage that, whenever relevant, you involve a statistician – again. You should of course have consulted one before you even started your research, but you will need to get another opinion before you proceed.

You should also clarify any ethical requirements that will be needed (see Figure 4.3). If you later find you have failed to comply with these ethical conditions, then you will have a major problem. Do not proceed in the hope that things will sort themselves out: if you have to admit that the project is flawed, now is the time to do so.

Some people find setting the brief extremely difficult. That's probably because, if done properly, it is difficult. But time spent on setting a sensible brief, and, in particular, on deciding in advance what message you choose to give (for examples, see Figure 3.5) will pay huge benefits later.

Before proceeding to Chapter 4, you should:
- have a clear brief, with written statements on the following:
  1 the message (one simple idea, with verb)
  2 the market
  3 the length
  4 the deadline
  5 the co-authors
- be familiar with your target journal's *Instructions to authors*.

4

Expand the brief

'I have now written my brief in the middle of a blank piece of paper . . .'

Gather your strength

This is a key moment. You may still be worrying that you have not made any progress, and that soon you are going to have to take the plunge and start writing. In fact, you are not merely over the worst, you have actually written your article. You have decided on the message. Admittedly, at this stage it consists of one idea and is 10–14 words long. But you have taken the all-important decision on what precisely, when all else is cut away (or lost in the mists of the reader's memory), you wish your reader to understand. You have also made the vital decision on where you will publish. You have defined your product, and now all you have to do is flesh it out.

There are two ways of proceeding. The first is the 'clerical' approach. This means going through all the material, in no particular order, pulling out bits of data, tables and references, and allocating them to one of the four boxes (Introduction, Methods, Results and Discussion) that make up the formal structure. This is a technique beloved of research junkies, who cannot stop seeking that crucial reference or extra fact, which they are convinced lies just around the corner.

This technique, however, will bring you up against one of the main problems in writing: it is easy to collect information to put in, but much harder to decide what to leave out. You can quickly fill each box to overflowing with potential material, but then you will have to do the literary equivalent of jumping up and down on the suitcase lid in a desperate bid to make sure that everything gets in. Which it won't.

The alternative approach is to make executive decisions and is dangerously close to what used to be called 'thinking'. It is based on the principle that you do not make a tree by shuffling all the twigs and leaves around. Instead you construct the trunk (the one-sentence message) and then work out the main branches you need (the themes of each paragraph). Note that these branches emerge from the trunk, and are not just tacked on to it. Note also that, once you have this broad framework in place, it is relatively straightforward to place the twigs. And even if you do put one or two in the wrong place, you will not have ruined the overall shape.

Look at the market requirements

Now take a rest from your own work and look at what the market demands. The form that your product must take has been tightly defined. Although there are some minor variations between journals, the main common requirements are sum-marised by the International Committee of Medical Journal Editors. This body grew out of a meeting of medical editors in Vancouver in 1978, and now is called the Vancouver Group. Its intention is to make life easier for authors and editorial staff by bringing in a common style. 'If authors prepare their manuscripts in the style specified in these requirements, editors of the participating journals will not return manuscripts for changes in style before considering them for publication.'

The group now meets regularly. More than 500 journals have agreed to follow their style, and they have also pronounced on other matters, such as order of authorship, patients' rights and conflict of interest. The fifth edition of the booklet *Uniform requirements for manuscripts submitted to biomedical journals* was published in 1997.[6] Before proceeding any further, therefore, familiarise yourself with these requirements over content.

These formal requirements will only give you part of the picture. I have analysed 89 pages appearing consecutively in the *BMJ* between October 1995 and March 1996, and also 50 pages in each of six different journals starting from June 1997. Clearly there are various structural features – such as type of opening, number of paragraphs in each section – that tend to vary according to the journal. Authors should therefore do some market research by finding copies of their target journal and carefully analysing (at this point) what appears in each of the four main sections. (Later on we will use the same type of market research to influence our decisions on the additional elements, such as the title and the references.)

Introduction

This section answers the question: why did we start? For the formal requirements see the Vancouver Group's instructions (Figure 4.1).

Figure 4.1: The Vancouver Group on the Introduction

State the purpose of the article and summarise the rationale for the study or observation. Give only strictly pertinent references and do not include data or conclusions from the work being reported.

The first paragraph(s) give the background to the paper. The real explanation for the paper (we got a grant, a patient turned up, or my professor wandered through one day with a pile of records . . .) may not always be appropriate. What you need to establish, usually through citing a small number of pertinent papers, is the gap in knowledge that your research is about to answer. Is it a new treatment for an old disease? Is it a challenge to orthodox procedures? Are you seeking a new piece of evidence that will solve a debate that has been raging for some time?

There is little scope to make the first sentence interesting: after all, the work, the findings and their implications all have to appear elsewhere. This is probably why most authors follow one of a small number of stock openings. Most give a brief lesson on the subject that is to be embarked upon (the 'seminar approach', see Figure 4.2):

> *Post-lunchtime amnesia in hospital doctors is charac-*
> *terised by a severe loss of memory one hour after consum-*
> *ing a meal of more than 87.3 calories taken between 12.10*
> *and 1.45.*

An alternative, favoured by *The Lancet*, is to emphasise the gravity of the condition (alarmist approach):

> *Post-lunchtime amnesia kills 3000 people a year in UK*
> *hospitals.*

A third technique is to refer to a controversy (Much Discussion Recently (MDR) approach):

> *There has been much discussion recently about the*
> *incidence and importance of post-lunchtime amnesia in*
> *hospital doctors.*

At the end of the Introduction, usually in the last sentence or paragraph, comes a brief sentence describing what the authors did.

> *The aim of this study was . . .*

or

> *We report . . .   We used data . . .   We have outlined . . .*

Figure 4.2: Types of first sentences in six different journals

	Seminar	Alarmist	MDR
N Engl J Med	45	2	3
*Lancet**	34	10	6
*BMJ**	37	4	9
J Ped	47	2	1
Ped Research	44	3	3
*Arch Dis Child**	43	4	3

*European-based.
Source: 50 consecutive articles from June 1, 1997.

The emergence of this key paragraph/sentence at the end of the introduction is an interesting development. In fact it could be used as an opening sentence for either the Introduction or the Discussion, but in its present form it acts as a hinge between the two sections.

Methods

This section answers the question: what did you do?

It expands on the information just given in the final paragraph of the Introduction. It should give readers enough information to enable them to evaluate, and in theory to replicate, the work. It should also explain the statistical methods and make it clear that ethical guidelines were followed. The formal requirements laid down by the Vancouver Group of editors are shown in Figure 4.3.

As a general principle, this section tells the story of what the authors did. Usually the best way to organise this will be in a logical framework of time.

Figure 4.3: The Vancouver Group on the Methods

Describe your selection of the observational or experimental subjects (patients or laboratory animals, including controls) clearly. Identify the age, sex and other important characteristics of the subjects. The definition and relevance of race and ethnicity are ambiguous. Authors should be particularly careful about using these categories.

Identify the methods, apparatus (manufacturer's name and address in parentheses) and procedures in sufficient detail to allow other workers to reproduce the results. Give references to established methods, including statistical methods; provide references and brief descriptions for methods that have been published but are not well known; describe new or substantially modified methods, give reasons for using them, and evaluate their limitations. Identify precisely all drugs and chemicals used, including generic name(s), dose(s) and route(s) of administration.

Reports of randomised clinical trials should present information on all major study elements including the protocol (study population, interventions or exposures, outcomes, and the rationale for statistical analysis), assignment of interventions (methods of randomisation, concealment of allocation to treatment groups), and the method of marking (blinding).

Authors submitting review manuscripts should include a section describing the methods used for locating, selecting, extracting and synthesising data. These methods should also be summarised in the abstract.

Ethics: When reporting experiments on human subjects, indicate whether the procedures followed were in accordance with the ethical standards of the responsible committee on human experimentation (institutional or regional) or with the Helsinki Declaration of 1975, as revised in 1983. Do not use patients' names, initials or hospital numbers, especially in illustrative material. When reporting experiments on animals, indicate whether the institution's or a national research council's guide for, or any national law on, the care and use of laboratory animals was followed.

Statistics: Describe statistical methods with enough detail to enable a knowledgeable reader with access to the original data to verify the reported results. When possible, quantify findings and present them with appropriate indicators of measurement error or uncertainty (such as confidence intervals). Avoid sole reliance on statistical hypothesis testing, such as the use of P values, which fails to convey important quantitative information. Discuss the eligibility of experimental subjects. Give details about randomisation. Describe the methods for and success of any blinding of observations. Report complications of treatment. Give numbers of observations. Report losses to observations (such as dropouts from a clinical trial). References for the design of the study and statistical methods should be to standard works when possible (with pages stated) rather than to papers in which the designs or methods were originally reported. Specify any general use computer programs used.

Results

This section answers the question: what did you find?

For most papers the heart of this section is the data, presented as tables or figures. Most articles in the six journals studied had one or two figures, with typically more than double that number in *Pediatric Research* (see Figure 4.4). All six tended to have two or three tables. Full specifications for the tables and figures (Figures 4.5 and 4.6) can be found in the Vancouver stylebook.

Authors often find it difficult to decide what goes in a table and what in the text. The Vancouver Group says the text should 'emphasise or summarise only important observations' (Figure 4.7). In other words use it as a narrative, to tell the main elements of the story and to draw the reader's attention to some of the main features of the tables and figures. For example, why are all the figures identical in the fourth row, and why is the value in the third column extremely interesting?

Discussion

This section answers the question: what does it mean?

The first sentence is relatively straightforward and it summarises the main findings of the research: 'In this study we found that . . .'

What usually follows is a brief essay about their implications, what the Vancouver Group calls 'new and important aspects of the study and the conclusions that follow from them' (Figure 4.8).

Figure 4.4: Mean number of figures and tables in six different journals

	Figures	Tables
N Engl J Med	1.5 (±1.3)	3.4 (±1.2)
*Lancet**	1.7 (±2.2)	2.8 (±1.4)
*BMJ**	0.7 (±1.0)	3.0 (±1.4)
J Ped	1.8 (±1.6)	2.6 (±1.3)
Ped Research	3.8 (±2.0)	2.2 (±1.8)
*Arch Dis Child**	1.3 (±1.4)	2.2 (±1.6)

Numbers in parentheses are the standard deviations.
*European-based.
Source: 50 consecutive articles from June 1, 1997.

Figure 4.5: The Vancouver Group on tables

Type or print out each table double-spaced on a separate sheet. Do not submit tables as photographs. Number tables consecutively in the order of their first citation in the text and supply a brief title for each. Give each column a short or abbreviated heading. Place explanatory matter in footnotes, not in the heading. Explain in footnotes all nonstandard abbreviations that are used in each table. For footnotes use the following symbols:

*, †, ‡, §, ||, ¶, **, ††, ‡‡

Identify statistical measures of variations such as standard deviation and standard error of the mean.

Do not use internal horizontal and vertical rules.

Be sure that each table is cited in the text.

If you use data from another published or unpublished source, obtain permission and acknowledge fully.

The use of too many tables in relation to the length of the text may produce difficulties in the layout of pages. Examine issues of the journal to which you plan to submit your paper to estimate how many tables can be used per 1000 words of text.

The editor, on accepting a paper, may recommend that additional tables containing important backup data too extensive to publish be deposited with an archival service, such as the National Auxiliary Publication Service in the United States, or made available by the authors. In that event an appropriate statement will be added to the text. Submit such tables for consideration with the paper.

Figure 4.6: The Vancouver Group on illustrations (figures)

Submit the required number of complete sets of figures. Figures should be professionally drawn and photographed; freehand or typewritten lettering is unacceptable. Instead of original drawings, X-ray films and other material, send sharp, glossy, black and white photographic prints, usually 127 × 172 mm (5 × 7 inches), but no larger than 203 × 254 mm (8 × 10 inches). Letters, numbers, and symbols should be clear and even throughout and of sufficient size that when reduced for publication each item will still be legible. Titles and detailed explanations belong in the legends for illustrations, not on the illustrations themselves.

Each figure should have a label pasted on its back indicating the number of the figure, author's name, and top of the figure. Do not write on the back of figures or scratch or mark them by using paper clips. Do not bend figures or mount them on cardboard.

Photomicrographs should have internal scale markers. Symbols, arrows, or letters used in photomicrographs should contrast with the background.

If photographs of people are used, either the subjects must not be identifiable or their pictures must be accompanied by written permission to use the photographs . . .

Figures should be numbered consecutively according to the order in which they have been first cited in the text. If a figure has been published, acknowledge the original source and submit written permission from the copyright holder to reproduce the material. Permission is required irrespective of authorship or publisher, except for documents in the public domain.

For illustrations in colour, ascertain whether the journal requires colour negatives, positive transparencies, or colour prints. Accompanying drawings marked to indicate the region to be reproduced may be useful to the editor. Some journals publish illustrations in colour only if the author pays for the extra cost.

Figure 4.7: The Vancouver Group on the Results

Present your results in logical sequence in the text, tables, and illustrations. Do not repeat in the text all the data in the tables or illustrations; emphasise or summarise only important observations.

On statistics: 'Put a general description of methods in the Methods section. When data are summarised in the Results section, specify the statistical methods used to analyse them. Restrict tables and figures to those needed to explain the argument of the paper and to assess its support. Use graphs as an alternative to tables with many entries; do not duplicate data in graphs and tables. Avoid non-technical uses of technical terms in statistics, such as "random" (which implies a randomising device), "normal", "significant", "correlations" and "sample". Define statistical terms, abbreviations and most symbols.'

Figure 4.8: The Vancouver Group on the Discussion

Emphasise the new and important aspects of the study and the conclusions that follow from them. Do not repeat in detail data or other material given in the Introduction or the Results section. Include in the Discussion section the implications of the findings and their limitations, including implications for future research. Relate the observations to other relevant studies.

Link the conclusions with the goals of the study but avoid unqualified statements and conclusions not completely supported by the data. In particular, authors should avoid making statements on economic benefits and costs until their manuscript includes economic data and analyses. Avoid claiming priority and alluding to work that has not been completed. State new hypotheses when warranted, but clearly label them as such. Recommendations, when appropriate, may be included.

Are the findings reliable? What do they actually mean? Do they shed light on the points raised in the Introduction? Where do we go from here? Are there any implications for clinical practice or public policy?

Figure 4.9: Types of last sentences in six different journals

	Another Puzzle Solved	Perhaps Possibly	More Research is Indicated
N Engl J Med	27	17	6
Lancet*	19	21	10
BMJ*	22	16	12
J Ped	26	16	8
Ped Research	20	20	10
Arch Dis Child*	27	10	13

*European-based journals.

Source: 50 consecutive articles from June 1, 1997.

The last sentence is extremely important because this is where, in most papers published in reputable journals, the message will appear (Figure 4.9).

This is what I call the 'Another Puzzle Solved' ending:

We conclude that HIV infection leads to progressive immune deterioration and AIDS irrespective of clotting factor usage.

or

Physicians treating asthmatic patients should use a history of major tranquilliser use as a marker for identifying patients at high risk for the serious complications of asthma.

There are two other types of ending, though these were far less common. The first was 'More Research is Indicated', such as:

Our results emphasise the need for further studies.

or

The effectiveness of such interventions cannot be inferred from this observational study but requires verification in experimental trials.

The other was the 'Perhaps Possibly' last sentence, in which there were signs that the authors had made progress, but had tempered it with cautious phrases, such as:

> *It may depend on . . . is likely to . . . This may have important implications for prevention.*

One conclusion was carefully wrapped in negatives:

> *The unexpected risk connected with the use of . . . indicates that the routine use of . . . cannot be recommended.*

Think

When you are clear as to what is required, you can return to your own work. You need to expand on your message so that it starts to conform to these specifications. An excellent way forward is branching, brainstorming or mind-mapping,[7] techniques now widely encouraged in schools as a useful way of revising for examinations, and which allow you to think through and develop the message you have identified. One of the great advantages is that, at this stage, all your thoughts are valuable and you do not have to make any decisions.

You need a large blank piece of paper. Write down your message in the middle of the paper. Then write down the four main questions your paper will have to answer: Why did you start? What did you do? What did you find? What does it all mean? (Figure 4.10). Now allow your brain to examine, expand, question and (where possible) answer the questions, and write down the results of these thoughts. Circle them. Link them with other circles where appropriate. Do not stop to evaluate what you put down. Allow yourself ten minutes. Using an egg-timer may help; among other things it is heartening to realise how quickly time has passed.

The exercise should leave you with a piece of paper covered

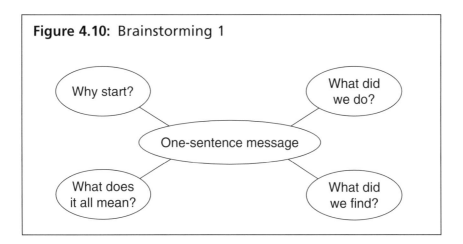

Figure 4.10: Brainstorming 1

with balloons (Figure 4.11), interlinked with lines and, per-haps, divided into larger balloons. You will have ensured that the main questions have been posed, and you will have a clear indication of what facts, opinions, references and other supporting material you will need to support them.

Use this technique to think about what you need to establish now that you have decided on your message. Some answers you will know already, others you will need to find out. But, by making the questions literally flow outwards from the brief, you are ensuring that you remain focused. Instead of trying to fit your information into the suitcase, you are preparing a list of what to pack.

Figure 4.11: Brainstorming 2: proposed article following analysis of 89 *BMJ* articles

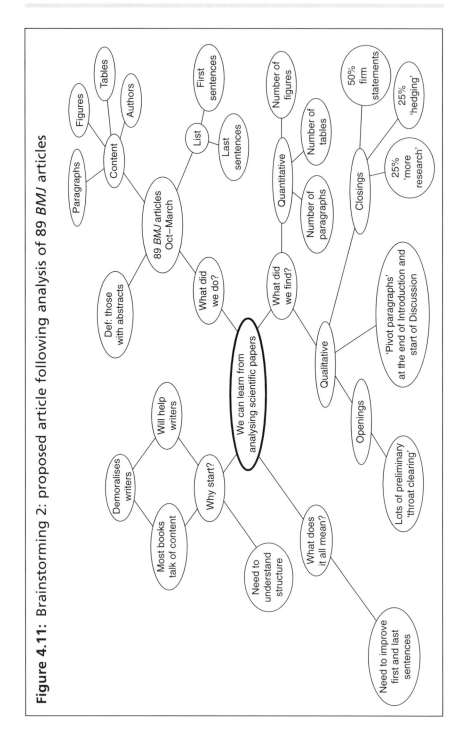

Before proceeding to Chapter 5, you should have:
- a clear grasp of the current requirements for each IMRAD section
- a large piece of paper containing the message – and the information needed to support that message.

BOOKCHOICE: What editors want

Hall G (ed) (1994) *How to Write a Paper* (2e). BMJ Publishing Group, London.

The value of this book is not so much that it shows people how to write (it doesn't) but it does show how those who judge writing currently think. The book consists of essays on various matters related to scientific publishing, mainly by clinicians who have also been editors. Despite its title, it is more concerned with the *what* than the *how*, and there is sometimes an engaging blend of pomposity and naiveté. There is a chapter on each IMRAD section, plus a stylish essay on style and useful insights into what a publisher does and the future of electronic publishing. The second edition contains chapters on two of the areas currently interesting editors – ethics and authorship.

Another change has been the chapter on the role of the manuscript assessor, which has now been written by Stephen G Spiro. As before in this section, the detailed advice given to assessors is useful because of the insights it provides into the market.

Introduction: '. . . There should be a succinct argument for the paper and some, not too much, justification, by referring to other related work in the field. Is there *really* the gap in knowledge that the authors claim, that is, is this a worthwhile project, irrelevant, or perhaps a reinvention of the wheel?'

Methods: '. . . very important and most reviewers make their decisions here. . . . the presentation, validation and extrapolation of the methods chosen have to be presented in such a way that they are clear, likely to be correct, and can be repeated elsewhere . . . The reviewer also needs to be satisfied that the number of subjects or tests performed are of sufficient magnitude or accuracy to give the result adequate statistical power . . .'

Results: '. . . should clearly summarise the relevant data. Many authors do this badly with much repetition in the text and often further repetition in the tables and figures . . .'

Discussion: '. . . unlikely to influence the decision to accept the paper. Nevertheless it is an important (section) and should clearly summarise the results, contain a critique of the methods used, comparisons with other work in the field, have a clear conclusion and, perhaps, pose questions for further work'.

In the first edition this section included this passage: 'A responsible editor will be aware that the editor is primarily interested in the "bottom line" – that is whether the manuscript should be accepted, returned to the author for revision, or rejected. In general, the assessor will make this assessment, which is highly subjective, on his or her "gut feeling" after reading the manuscript'. This advice has gone now, which is a pity.

5

Make a plan, or four

'Drawing a creative (non-linear) pattern is often useful for gathering ideas and as a start to the planning stage; converting this to a logical linear structure may be more difficult.'

Understanding structure

Your head should be bursting not only with details of the work you have done, but also of the requirements you have to meet. You now need to start making some decisions – but before you do so it is helpful to understand some of the elements of structure.

One of the common ways of talking about writing is in terms of total number of words. The problem is not the quantity of words, but how you order them.

A more sensible way forward is to think of the paragraph as the main unit. Each paragraph is a block of type that stands alone, and therefore it is sensible to assume that each covers a particular area. We can count up how many there are in a typical paper in our target journal, and (with the exception of the Methods section in highly scientific journals) the results are remarkably consistent (Figure 5.1). The following pattern would do for most journals.

- Introduction – 2 paragraphs
- Methods – 6 paragraphs
- Results – 6 paragraphs
- Discussion – 7 paragraphs.

This immediately makes things easier – we have 21 units of thought to prepare.

Figure 5.1: Mean number of paragraphs per section in six different journals

	Introduction	Methods	Results	Discussion
N Engl J Med	2.6 ($\pm$1.1)	9.2 ($\pm$3.3)	8.9 ($\pm$3.8)	6.9 ($\pm$1.8)
Lancet*	2.6 ($\pm$1.3)	7.6 ($\pm$3.6)	6.1 ($\pm$2.9)	7.0 ($\pm$2.6)
BMJ*	2.3 ($\pm$0.9)	6.0 ($\pm$3.7)	5.9 ($\pm$3.1)	7.4 ($\pm$2.8)
J Ped	2.6 ($\pm$1.1)	6.7 ($\pm$3.4)	7.0 ($\pm$3.9)	7.3 ($\pm$2.8)
Ped Research	3.0 ($\pm$1.3)	9.6 ($\pm$3.8)	6.3 ($\pm$2.9)	8.5 ($\pm$3.4)
Arch Dis Child*	2.7 ($\pm$1.3)	6.5 ($\pm$4.0)	6.1 ($\pm$4.0)	6.9 ($\pm$2.8)

Numbers in parentheses are the standard deviations.
*European-based journals.
Source: 50 consecutive articles from June 1, 1997.

Now we know roughly how many paragraphs to put in each section, we need to consider how we should construct each paragraph. The trick is to realise that there are two types of sentences. Go through a piece of text and underline or highlight the key sentences so that you are left with a much smaller version than your original text. This has divided your sentences into two types. The 'key' sentences – those that you have underlined – move the argument forwards. The 'supporting' sentences – those not underlined – illustrate and support your arguments.

Should the 'key' sentences appear at the beginning of each

paragraph or at the end? Scientists tend to structure all their writing in the style of IMRAD. Thus:

It is well documented that fires in nightclubs are a major hazard [Introduction]. Last night I went to a fire that took place in a nightclub in the middle of town and spoke to the senior fire officer [Methods]. He told me that 87 people perished [Results]. It is believed that fewer people would have died had the fire exits not been locked [Discussion].

The alternative is to start with the most important piece of information, then elaborate, explain and, if necessary, prove. This is commonly used by professional communicators, who call it (probably inaccurately from the mathematical point of view) the inverted triangle. Thus:

Eighty-seven people have perished in a fire because all the emergency exits were locked. It happened in a nightclub in the centre of town shortly after midnight last night. The number of deaths was confirmed to me by the senior fire officer at the scene.

Your paragraphs will work well, and keep the reader interested, if you write them so that they become in effect a series of inverted triangles. Put the key sentence at the beginning of the paragraph, as, for instance:

'We then selected the patients . . .'

'Once we had selected the patients we gave them a battery of tests . . .'

'There are three reasons why our findings are of interest . . .'

then support and elaborate, as necessary. This has important implications for the planning of an article. If you can take out all but the key sentences after you have written, then obviously you can plan by deciding what these key sentences will cover.

Making a plan (or rather four)

The position so far is as follows. You have formulated your one-sentence message and decided on your market. You have revisited your data and rearranged it according to the four main questions that you need to answer. You know that you need to end up with four pieces of writing of, say, two paragraphs, four paragraphs, four paragraphs and five paragraphs.

Keep well away from your data, but take with you the

Figure 5.2: Plan of article reporting results of post-lunchtime amnesia in hospital doctors survey

Introduction

Deep concern over post-lunchtime amnesia (PLA)
Survey of hospital doctors to discover prevalence

Methods/what we did

Sample
Questionnaire
Procedure
Statistical analysis

Results

General prevalence
Surgeons vs physicians
Links with gender
Links with medical school

Discussion/what we found

Much higher than expected and probably related to medical school
Obvious need for treatment
But treatment some way in the future
New directions for research
Need for education

Message: We need to make more people aware of the dangers of PLA.

jottings you made at the end of the last chapter. Using these as a guide, construct your four plans (Figure 5.2).

Restrict your plan to brief ideas or subject headings only. The purpose of this stage is to build the branches of your tree. In other words chart your argument. If you do not keep away from the details at this stage they will probably swamp you.

At the end of this chapter you should have:
- four simple plans, one for each of the four sections: Introduction, Methods, Results, Discussion.

6

Write the first draft

'The hardest part of anything I write is always the introduction. I can spend days thinking of a good opening sentence.'

Conquer the fear of writing . . .

The next part of the process is to start the actual writing. This should be fun, but seems to traumatise most people. They go to severe lengths to avoid it, and use various strategies such as hunting references, making coffee, telephoning unloved relatives or sitting for hours in front of a blank screen, blankly.

I blame the educationists, who have so brainwashed us that we cannot undertake a writing task without believing that it is an examination. But writing for a journal is not that kind of test. What is being judged is not what writers have happened to learn (or remember), but the particular contribution to knowledge that they are describing. It is not a time trial and what is important is not the first draft but the final version.

Understanding this should help to make this part of the writing process much less frightening. Putting the words down on paper becomes not an end point, but a beginning. This should be a time of creativity, not criticism (see Bookchoice, p. 58). If you have done the preparatory thinking, all the information and arguments are already lodged in your head;

you now have to unlock them. What you write will not be perfect, but at this stage it doesn't matter.

Get ready to write

You need three things only for the writing process: a clear plan, a suitable writing implement and peace and quiet.

A clear plan

Take only your plan with you into this stage. Do not surround yourself with all the raw material, such as tables and references and longhand notes of seminar papers. It matters little at this stage whether your experiment killed 43 rats or 47; you will know that, since there were only 50, the trend was to die. Go for the flow; you can add the details later.

A suitable writing implement

Most people write directly on to a word processor of some kind. This can be fast and enjoyable, but there are two main problems. First, you may be tempted to go back and fiddle with words and phrases. Second, you may be tempted to go back and fiddle with whole paragraphs. If you can resist such temptations, word processors are now a sensible option.

Some writers feel that using a dictating machine is cheating, but it has the advantage that you can swiftly put down a first draft. If you have someone who can then transcribe it for you, this is a painless way to start. You will be speaking aloud, and so are more likely to use the rhythms and vocabulary of oral speech (which is much easier to unravel than that which presently goes under the title of Proper Scientific Writing). Unfortunately, it can be too easy to get carried away with the sound of your own voice. If you choose this option, make sure that you keep your plan in a convenient place. And that you keep referring to it.

Others prefer more traditional methods, such as a pen or pencil. These are relatively slow (and perhaps painful), but you can still do 30–40 words a minute if you write without stopping. Some swear that a fountain pen gives them the right speed. Others insist on a pencil with a rubber but, to stop you fiddling rather than writing, I would recommend cutting off the rubber.

Peace and quiet

Many people say that finding time is the major problem. They are extremely busy people (parents, lovers, doctors, scientists, model aeroplane society secretaries), and even when they manage to find time, either at home or at work, other people constantly interrupt them.

The answer is not to see when you can block off 2–3 hours of uninterrupted time; that is almost impossible these days. Instead try to snatch 20 minutes a day. For reasons that I am about to explain, that should be enough to write about 700 words. Four such snatches, and you will have completed the first draft of the paper. This is a controversial assertion, but, if true, think of how it will revolutionise your life. (As supporting evidence I can state that in 20 minutes I managed to write the first 720 words of the first draft of this chapter.)

Go with the flow

The key is to be creative, not critical, and to turn the first draft from a penance into a festival. It should be fun.

At this stage you need big ideas and logical flow. You are the expert on the subject you have chosen. You also have a plan to remind you of the steps you have decided to take. Flesh these out: your goal is to end up with the outline of each section. There will almost certainly be gaps, but you can fill these later.

So, when you start to write, write down the first sentence immediately. If it isn't the perfect opening sentence (and it is unlikely that it will be) start with the second sentence. Or go back and take a run at the start with sentences that can easily be dismantled later, such as:

I am about to sit here for 20 minutes and write about the wonderful experiment I have just completed. What we did was . . .

When you have finished one sentence, go on to the next. When you have finished that one, go on again. And so on. Do not under any circumstances look back.

Use your natural language. Do not try to imitate the style of your chosen journal at this stage. Do not try to impress your professor. Instead, imagine that you are speaking to an informed colleague over a beer or coffee. Use the language with which you are most comfortable and you will probably find that it will end up much clearer than if you were consciously constructing individual sentences for publication. You may have to translate this later into the dull style favoured by your target journal, but that will be easy.

If your first language is not English, consider writing the first draft in your own language. At this stage we are talking about thought processes; an appropriate language can easily come later.

Whatever language you choose, by the end of 20 minutes or so (and again you may wish to put a timer on) you will have made considerable progress. You will have some words on paper and those words will have taken a shape.

Some people will never believe that writing in short bursts will solve their problems. They tend to be those who, as soon as they have written one sentence, will go back and worry about it. They constantly fiddle with the meaning, checking whether the references are exactly right, or looking up obscure points of punctuation in a heavy tome on grammar. Let them enjoy this process if they want – but it will reduce rather than increase their chances of getting published.

Write each section in turn

I prefer writing the sections in the order in which they will be read. This seems to be a logical way of doing things, and enables me to keep focused. I know that many people recommend that you should start with the Methods section on the grounds that this is an easy place to start. If that works for you, do it.

Overcoming writer's block

From time to time you will find it impossible to get going, or you will simply dry up. This is commonly called writer's block. It can be nature's way of telling you that you are bored – in which case the solution is simple: do something else. Most people have their times when they seem to write best: work out when yours is. If you cannot force the pace at other times, don't feel guilty. Stop.

However, writer's block can also be your subconscious mind's way of telling you that your writing has lost its way. In this case it is also time to call a temporary halt. You might wish to talk to a colleague. If that fails to work, walk away from the article, take a good rest, and then think out the brief again. You should have already spotted if you were persevering with the unpublishable, so the worst possible scenario is that you will have to start again from scratch. Since you have done most of the research, that will take much less time than you will think, and certainly will cost much less time than if you continue on your fruitless task.

Before proceeding to Chapter 7, you should have:
- four rough drafts of the Introduction, Methods, Results and Discussion.

BOOKCHOICE: Writing without pain and guilt

Klauser HA (1987) *Writing on Both Sides of the Brain*. HarperCollins, San Francisco.

This is a gem of a book, despite its somewhat gushing tone. It is more than 10 years old now, but still listed at bookshops. I have not yet found another book that deals so well with the various *processes* involved in writing.

It is full of sensible advice that should leave you motivated to start – and, more importantly, finish – your next writing task. The key notion is the division of our brains into two sides, and with it the division of writing into two functions – the critical and the creative (or what Klauser calls, after characters in *The Tempest*, Caliban and Ariel). We need both – but not at the same time.

From this comes a number of excellent ideas:

- start a log so that you can write about your writing – what you are achieving and where your problems lie
- consider your rumination time an essential part of writing
- when writing and thinking about writing, try to go that extra bit further (what she calls 'hitting the wall')
- write without judging what you are writing (i.e. give yourself 'permission to write garbage')
- start writing first thing in the morning . . .

As Klauser says, the book is for you 'if you are tired of putting off the writing that needs to be done, if you believe that you have an idea locked up inside of you that you lack the confidence to share in writing, if you are holding yourself back from getting a promotion because you are not doing the writing that your chosen profession calls for . . .' It certainly altered my own views.

7

Rewrite your draft

'Checking for grammar, style and consistency is vital. How can we rely on the accuracy of a scientist's work if he/she shows no accuracy in his/ her use of language?'

Now comes the pain . . .

Once you have finished your first draft, walk away from it. Leave it for a time: some people say for a few days, but this may not always be practicable. The important thing is to put some distance between you and it, so you will be able to approach it with some objectivity, and not see it as a part of your soul that others tamper with at their peril.

When you return, brace yourself for some hard work. Some people complain that they spend too much time rewriting. I suspect that they are still hung up on the feeling that they must get it right first time. The real test of a piece of writing is not how quickly it was written, but whether it works for the target audience. To complain that you have a writing problem because you took 12 or so drafts for an article that was published in *Nature* is missing the point. As with all products, the secret to success is hard work; if something looks polished, the chances are that someone has spent a lot of time doing the polishing.

Sometimes things do go wrong, however, and you find that

you are getting nowhere: the last eight drafts, for instance, may have taken you back to where you started some weeks ago. There are ways of limiting such disasters. First, keep to your deadlines, which will cut down your inclination to fiddle for the sake of fiddling. Second, for at least some of the time, rewrite on hard copy rather than on screen, which again will reduce the opportunity for uncontrolled fiddling. Third, have clear in your own mind the criteria you will use for judging what you have written, and how you will go about applying them.

As a start, I recommend dividing this process into two: macroediting and microediting.

Macroediting

Print out your first draft and read it privately. You do not need a pencil at this stage. Try not to worry if the words are misspelt (as some of them certainly will be). Read the article through quickly to get some impression of how it looks now that it has moved from your head on to a piece of paper. Then start asking yourself the difficult questions.

Is there a clear message?

What was the message you chose to write about? Where does it appear? Will it be clear to your chosen readers (i.e. the editor and reviewers)? Is what you set out to say the same as what you have written? Or have some changes of emphasis crept in? Is your message clearly positioned in the last sentence of the Discussion? Now that the message is in black and white, does it still look worth saying?

These are central questions. No matter how polished your prose, publication is unlikely unless you are saying something worthwhile. Remember the definition in Chapter 1: scientific papers should be original and important. Now that your paper is beginning to take shape on paper – is it?

Do you prove your message?

Given that you have a clear message in place, do you prove it? Is the evidence clearly stated, and well supported? If you were your own worst enemy (or competing against yourself for a job) how would you criticise the article?

Is it right for the market you have chosen?

Does the article meet the general requirements laid down in the *Instructions to authors*, in particular the length. Do you have a reasonable number of paragraphs? Does the style conform to the style of the journal? Is it in tune with the editor's view of the readership. Here you will find one of the various 'readability' scores a useful tool for your market research (Figure 7.1).

Is the structure appropriate and reader-friendly?

Have you kept to the required IMRAD structure? Look at each section. Does the Introduction really explain why you started and does the last sentence describe what you did? Does the Methods section go on to describe this in detail? Does the Results section reveal what you found? And does the Discussion section start with a sentence summarising what you found, then go on to consider the most important implications?

Figure 7.1: Gunning Fog Score[8]

There are several tests of whether a piece of writing is likely to be easily readable or not, and the one I favour was that devised in the early 1940s by Professor Gunning in the United States. It is based on the assumption that the longer the words and the longer the sentences, then the harder a piece of writing is likely to be.

The index is calculated using the following steps.

1 Count up a passage of about 100 words, ending in a full stop.
2 Calculate the average sentence length by dividing 100 by the number of sentences.
3 Count the number of long words, defined as words of three syllables or more, but excluding:
   • two-syllable verbs that become three by 'ed' or 'ing' (e.g. committed, committing)
   • proper nouns, like Winchester or Canterbury or Germany or Italy
   • two common short words used together, such as photo-copy
   • jargon that readers will know (be very careful with inter-preting this).
4 Add the average sentence length to the number of long words.
5 Multiply by 0.4. That is the reading score.

Typical scores: Airport novel 6; tabloid newspapers 8–10; middlebrow newspapers 10–12; serious newspapers 12–14; medical journals 14–16; insurance company small print 20.

Examples

'In conclusion, our data support the hypothesis that non-steroidal anti-inflammatory drug use protects against the devel-opment of colorectal neoplasia./ The strength of the association is similar to that found in the three other epidemiological stud-ies in which non-steroidal anti-inflammatory drug use has been associated with a halving of the risk of colorectal cancer./ Studies are now needed to confirm these findings, to determine how non-steroidal anti-inflammatory drugs might act, and

Figure 7.1 (*continued*)

particularly to see if non-steroidal anti-inflammatory drugs
can prevent the recurrence of adenoma or even cause sporadic
adenomas to regress.' (*BMJ*, Friday 20 July, 1993)

'Aspirin, once seen as a humble household remedy for head-
aches, may also protect against bowel cancer as well as helping
with arthritis and reducing the risk of heart disease and strokes,
says a report in the *BMJ* today./ The study was done by Dr
Richard Logan and colleagues from the University of Notting-
ham Medical School./ They say that those who took aspirin or
other non-steroidal anti-inflammatory drugs (NSAIDs) had half
the risk of developing the pre-cancerous lumps which go on to
become bowel cancer as non-takers./ In some cases the dose was
as low as half an aspirin a day.'

	BMJ	Guardian
1 Number of sentences	3	4
2 Average sentence length	33	25
3 Long words	24	9
4 2 + 3	57	34
5 Fog Score ($\times$ 0.4)	22.8	13.6

The index does not predict good writing, so artificially
manipulating it won't automatically turn something unreadable
into something that is easy to read. But it does seem to
correlate with readable writing.

There is no such thing as a 'good' or 'bad' score in isolation.
The most important thing is that the score of your text should
match the score of your market. When writing for a particular
journal, take a selection of articles and do a Fog Score on them.
Yours should be a comparable score.

The test can also give useful information if there is a
particular writing problem. For instance, one student was sent
on a course on the grounds that she was a bad writer. Doing
the test on her writing and on the writing of her professor
showed that she was writing to a score of 12 (quite reasonable)
while the professor favoured a tortuous style of 18.

Figure 7.2: The yellow marker test

The 'yellow marker' test can identify the underlying structure of an article. Go through with a marker pen and highlight those sentences that you feel are absolutely essential. This should leave you with a much shorter but still understandable version. This should show you the 'key' and 'supporting' sentences – plus the underlying structure of the writing.

Look at where these sentences fall. If most of the highlighted sentences come at the beginning of each paragraph, you will have a solid and easy-to-follow structure. If you have paragraphs with no sentences highlighted, then ask: is that paragraph necessary? If you have highlighted several sentences together, ask: are you risking information overload? If the highlighted sentence is buried in the middle of a paragraph, ask: would it work better at the beginning?

Do the yellow marker test (Figure 7.2). Have you met the requirements of the IMRAD structure? Does the last paragraph of the Introduction state clearly what you did, and the first paragraph of the Conclusion state clearly your main findings? Do your key sentences come at the start of each paragraph? Do your paragraphs follow on from each other in a sensible fashion?

Work on the opening sentence. As a general rule, this is particularly dull, so now is your chance to make it more attractive (or rather, less dull) (Figure 7.3). Now look to your final sentence. Are you asking for more research? Are you being needlessly tentative about what you have found? Or have you a straightforward sentence showing exactly what contribution you have made to our knowledge?

These macroediting questions are important. But many people neglect them, probably because it is a lot easier to move commas around or repeat the rules of long-gone grammar teachers. Be patient: once you have asked the big question – and provided adequate solutions – you can start playing with the details.

Figure 7.3: First six words test

Conventions of a scientific paper dictate that the first sentence of a scientific paper gives the background to the 'story' rather than (as with mainstream journalism) the essence of that story. But within that constraint there is plenty of scope for making the first sentence more – or less – interesting.

You can test your own first sentence by counting out the first six words of your article. Why six words? It is to some extent arbitrary, but it gives the writer enough time to establish the subject and the reader enough words to establish if he or she will be interested. And it can be revealing, as shown in the following examples all taken from original papers published in the *BMJ* between October 1995 and March 1996.

In several articles the first six words were empty words or padding – 'throat clearing' – that could profitably have been removed, such as:

It has been suggested that up . . .

It is generally accepted that the . . .

There has been much discussion recently . . .

Other sentences started with precise – but not important – details that would have been better left until later in the sentence, or paragraph:

On 24 and 25 June 1995 . . .

Since the late 1960s most public . . .

In the Netherlands the prevention of . . .

The following sentences, on the other hand, work much better. The subject of the sentence (and of the article itself) is early in the first sentence. They are therefore far more likely to grab and keep the interest:

Wine has an ancient reputation for . . .

Insulin dependent diabetes develops on the . . .

Oral contraceptives have been linked with . . .

Most low birthweight babies have a . . .

Microediting

Omssions and errors

Now is the time to check on your facts. Go back to your 'raw material'. Was it 1349 or 1347 rats that died? Have you allowed a decimal point to move? (When talking about doses, for instance, this could literally be a fatal mistake.) Are all your numbers consistent? 7 + 5 + 12 does not come to 23, and 7 is 29.1% not 21.9% of that total. Was that important paper published by Smith, Smith and Jones on page 1147, or by Smith, Jones and Smith on page 1174?

Be obsessive. Nothing will ruin your hard work more quickly and more effectively than the discovery, after publication, that there are several inaccuracies that could (or should) have been avoided.

Many journals provide checklists: this is the time to use them. There are various agreed principles, such as the Consort statement on randomised clinical trials.[9] Read them and check that you comply.

Spelling and grammar

Most computers have a spell check. Use it. It will take minutes rather than hours, and you will almost certainly pick up one or two misspellings that you have not and (since you wrote them in the first place) probably will never spot. (For instance, did you notice the missing *i* in *omissions* above?) Spell checks, however, are fallible and will not alert you to good words in the wrong place, as in: *Two bee whore knot two bee . . .*

Grammar will give you many more problems, mainly because it has become a battleground for those who wish to score points and assert that they have had a better education. These people cite certain 'rules' that they learnt at school, and scream with delight whenever you break one of them. In general these rules are limited to the following:

1 do not start a sentence with And or But
2 don't split an infinitive
3 don't end with a preposition.

Unfortunately for these critics, most contemporary authorities say that these rules are now outdated. *The Good English Guide* says this about split infinitives: 'If you don't want to upset anyone, you will avoid split infinitives. If you care more about writing good clear English, you will be prepared to *fearlessly split* any infinitive to allow words to fall naturally'.[10] Gowers is clear about starting a sentence with 'But': 'The idea is now dead'.[11]

We should not slavishly follow rules that have passed their natural shelf-life. Nor should we feel inferior in education or ability if we didn't happen to attend a school that gave formal grammar classes. Nevertheless, we do need to follow the main grammatical rules if we wish to make ourselves understood. One solution is to use one of the many software packages that have grammar checks. Unfortunately these take a long time to run, and are of limited value if, for instance, they keep telling you that you are breaking a rule of which you are completely ignorant.

My own recommendations are:

1 invest in a good but short book (see Bookchoice p. 74)
2 find a friend who knows about grammar (but preferably a stylist rather than a pedant)
3 read your own words carefully, and apply common sense.

You do not need to define a dangling modifier to realise that there is something wrong with the following:

Having vomited all night, the doctor visited the patient with a bowl.

Style – in theory

There is a distinguished tradition in English writing, from George Orwell and Somerset Maugham to Philip Howard and Keith Waterhouse – that firmly equates style with energy, clarity and simplicity. Editors of scientific journals adhere to these principles, as do those who write on scientific writing.

Nearly 60 years ago *The Lancet's Instructions to Authors* stated: 'Every sentence should be as simple as possible: apart from technical terms it should be intelligible at a first reading to any educated person. The pompous circumlocution often thought appropriate to scientific publications is an enemy to clear thinking and an obstacle to the spread of information among busy practitioners.[12] In 1996 the authors of *Successful Scientific Writing* expressed a similar view: 'A scientific paper should hold the attention of its readers by the importance of its content, not by its literary presentation. For this reason, the simplest writing style is usually best. This does not mean that you should avoid technical words . . . What it does mean is that you should not include verbose words and phrases in a vain attempt to impress the reader with your intellect and scientific status'.[13]

Every year more books are published with similar sentiments, accompanied by long lists of how to acquire a good style. More are coming out as I write. In view of the fact that the publication of these instructions has had absolutely no effect so far, I would suggest that you should merely ask the following three questions. Dealing with them sensibly will improve your prose considerably.

1 Are any sentences too long? One of the most common ways in which writing goes wrong is when sentences are too long. The Fog Test (Figure 7.1) suggests that we should be getting

4–5 sentences every 100 words (which is not the same as saying all sentences should be 20–25 words long). If the length starts to rise towards and beyond 30 words, then you could be heading for trouble.

One common fault is to start with a subordinate phrase or clause, or even two:

> *Since long term survival seems to be similar after initial resuscitation, whether this occurs in or outside hospital (81% over two years), any improvement in the success of cardiopulmonary resuscitation outside hospital would be beneficial.*

Then there is the reverse hamburger of a sentence, where the meat is ruined by a soggy mass in the middle:

> *The development of vaccines against infection with hepatitis B, initially by purification of the virus surface protein from the plasma of carriers and more recently via its synthesis in yeast by using recombinant DNA technology, has enabled the chain of infection to be broken.*

Finally comes the overload:

> *When only gastroscopy requests meant to exclude malignancy are tolerated, an adequate prediction model for peptic ulcer, or using a serologic test for further selection, not only helps by reducing the number of gastroscopy requests for other reasons, but also might support the decision to prescribe H_2-receptor antagonists before ordering further diagnostic tests.*

In this case, the best thing is to start again, perhaps by trying to tell a colleague what you are trying to say. You might find it helpful to do this in the pub, or a similar social setting.

2 Are there any passives that would be better in the active voice? The best way to start a sentence in English is with the subject:

> *As concern about the impact of current economic conditions on public health was shown by a substantial number of epidemiologists, the main activity was still investigation of medical priorities in the light of a background of decreasing wealth and employment opportunities*

can become:

> *Many epidemiologists were worried about the impact of current economic conditions on public health. They therefore concentrated on investigating medical priorities amid a background of decreasing wealth and employment opportunities.*

Richard Smith, editor of the *BMJ*, is clear which version he would prefer: 'The tragedy of scientific writing is that whole generations of young people who started writing:

> *The cat sat on the mat* and *Mummy is eating an orange*

have been forced to write:

> *The mat is sat on by the cat*

and:

> *The orange is being eaten by Mummy*

because it is more scientific. Nobody knows why it is supposed to be more scientific, but I imagine that it has something to do with the objectivity of science'.[14]

What he means is many scientists still insist that the passive is more objective, a concept that I find difficult to accept.

> *The passive is preferred*

illustrates the main problem: who is doing the preferring? The writer? The writer and his friends? Most people? A lot of people? There is a lack of clarity, which is absent in the following active versions:

I prefer the passive, or *Many scientists who were at school before the 1960s prefer the passive.*

3 Are there long words that could be replaced with shorter ones? Long words are not a sign of cleverness. Scientists may feel they have to use *approximately* rather than *about*, but in no sense is the latter less scientific. Taken to extremes, a sentence such as:

We would not have enough hospital beds if there were a major asthma epidemic

becomes:

Once a designated hospital is saturated, patients are diverted to supporting hospitals; but this option would not be available in a large epidemic of asthma if all hospitals in an area were affected.

The answer is straightforward: be vigilant. To help in this task I have a list of ten commonly used pompous words and phrases, with their shorter alternatives (Figures 7.4 and 7.5). Eliminating these would be a start.

Figure 7.4: Ten pompous words to avoid and suggested alternatives

additional	more
approximately	about
assistance	help
elevated	raised, higher
frequently	often
following	after
novel	new
participate	take part
possesses	has
sacrifice	kill

Figure 7.5: Ten pompous phrases to avoid and suggested alternatives

affect in a positive way	benefit
a number of	many
at this point in time	now
due to the fact that	because
in addition to	also
in the event of	if
prior to	before
male paediatric patient	boy
upper limbs	arms
subsequent to	after

Style – in practice

Clearly there is a huge gap between what the writing 'experts' advocate, and what happens in practice (Figure 7.6). The above guidelines are by no means drastic, and applying them should make any piece of writing far more accessible and easy to read. But anyone reading a journal will appreciate that even these basic principles are often ignored.

Figure 7.6: Copy-editing in practice

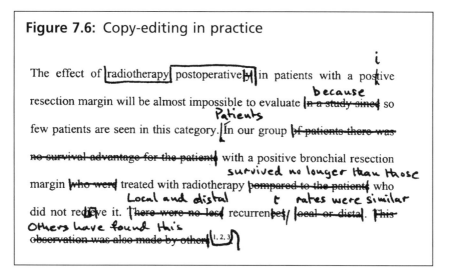

This can be very confusing for inexperienced writers. From time to time a participant comes to the second day of a training course saying that he or she has written simply, as we suggested, only to find that the professor has changed it all back on the grounds that it was not 'proper scientific writing'.

Fortunately there is a simple resolution to this problem. For this kind of writing, style is not, and should not be, a way in which we express our personalities. (If you want to do that, try poetry.) It is the way we get information across from one person to another. In this context, style becomes the choice of words and constructions most likely to get the message across to the target audience. This means that the most valuable – indeed the only – criterion of whether a style is 'right' or 'good' is to ask the question: is it appropriate for the target journal?

This in turn means that you should look carefully at the papers it publishes, analyse the kind of language and the kind of sentences that are used, and write in that style.

This, of course, is a rational and sensible view. You are about to find that the debate over style becomes a major battleground as your colleagues and your superiors insist that their views are 'better' than yours. What you write will almost certainly be changed, and not always for the best. Try not to waste time getting drawn into what is really quite unimportant detail. Above all, don't take it personally.

> Before proceeding to Chapter 8, you should have:
> - a manuscript that you feel is ready to be shown to others.

BOOKCHOICE: What is a 'good' style?

Goodman NW and Edwards MB (1997) *Medical Writing: a prescription for clarity* (2e). Cambridge University Press, Cambridge.

There are many books on how to write in a 'good' scientific style, and many of them say the same thing. They wheel out endless lists of what to avoid, such as long sentences, pompous words and the passive voice. Curiously, these lists seem to have made no difference whatsoever, and daily we see a sharp increase in the volume of papers published in a badly written and often unintelligible style.

Aspiring writers should read at least one of these books, and I would recommend *Medical Writing: a prescription for clarity*. It is now in its second edition, with a new chapter on clear graphs, new exercises – and slightly fewer cartoons. It remains a model of what it pleads for – 'clear, simple unambiguous writing'. The authors have no time for the arguments that are constantly used, such as writing should be allowed to reflect personality and long words are somehow more scientific.

'Bad writing is contagious if the reader has not received an adequately immunising dose of good', they say. And they advocate some good general principles:

- prefer familiar nouns
- use short words in short sentences
- get at least two people to read what you have written
- read books about English.

They add plenty of the usual detailed advice on commonly misspelt words, imprecise words, superfluous phrases and pompous words (from the usual *commence* and *administer* to the more sophisticated snobbisms such as *adumbrate*).

The most useful part of the book is the excellent examples that the reader can try to improve. In some cases, the authors offer their own solutions, as in:

> *At the junction of sutures and staples, however, a meaningful comparison was thereby available. Further, by randomisation of the distribution, a more extensive appraisal of the scar was made*

which becomes:

> *We could compare sutures and staples where they were next to one another, and increase the validity of the comparison by randomising their distribution!*

The authors are clear that they wish to 'encourage good writing by examining bad writing', and this they clearly do. Read and enjoy the book. Buy it for others. And try not to be too depressed as you see others not simply ignore its advice, but also argue vehemently in favour of all that the book has demolished.

8

Prepare the additional elements

'Colleagues who write, but are not professional writers, frequently fail to see the need to revise – with predictable results.'

The article itself – the text from first word to last – is now complete. Check that its layout meets the requirements of your target journal (Figure 8.1).

Now start working on the additional elements that the market requires, such as title, abstracts, key words and list of references. Follow the same principle as you would follow if designing a label for a sauce bottle: do not invest time in the task until you are satisfied that you have the basic ingredients right.

Do not expect these tasks to be squeezed in somehow. Doing them properly will take several hours and you should allow for this in advance.

The title page

This task may seem simple. On the face of it, all you have to do is put down on one sheet of paper who wrote what (Figure 8.2).

Figure 8.1: The Vancouver Group on preparation of manuscript

Type or print out the manuscript on white bond paper, 216 × 279 mm (8.5 × 11 inches), or ISO A4 (212 × 297 mm), with margins of at least 25 mm (1 inch). Type or print on only one side of the paper. Use double spacing throughout, including for the title page, abstract, text, acknowledgements, references, individual tables, and legends. Number pages consecutively, beginning with the title page. Put the page number in the upper or lower right-hand corner of each page.

Manuscripts on disks – For papers that are close to final acceptance, some journals require authors to provide a copy in electronic form (on a disk); they may accept a variety of word-processing formats or text (ASCII) files. When submitting disks, authors should:

- be certain to include a printout of the version of the article that is on the disk
- put only the latest version of the manuscript on the disk
- name the file clearly
- label the disk with the format and the file name
- provide information on the hardware and software used.

Yet this page will probably cause more trouble than any other single page. The requirements are as follows.

The title

This causes an inordinate amount of pain and suffering, probably because it is written in larger letters. Authors and co-authors often become enveloped in the most horrendous rows, even though a paper will almost certainly never be rejected for its title: if the editor doesn't like it, he will change it.

The problem is that there is no consensus on what makes a good title. The Vancouver Group says it should be 'concise and informative', which is fine as far as it goes, which isn't very far. If you look in a number of journals, you will see a variety of

Figure 8.2: Title Page

**Prevalence of post-lunchtime amnesia among doctors
in UK hospitals: results of a cross-sectional survey**

Andrew W Smith MB BS[1], William AW Smith MD MRCP[1], Emily S
Dupont BSc M Phil[2]

1 Department of Prandiology, New University of Middleshire,
Middleshire, UK
2 Institut Alimentaire, Paris 23, France

Address for correspondence: Dr AW Smith, Room 321, Department
of Prandiology, New University of Middleshire, Middleshire, UK

This research was undertaken with a grant of £100,000 from the
Obecalp Foundation

Running head: Prevalence of PLA in UK hospital doctors

different styles. Some editors like a string of words: *The prevalence of post-lunchtime amnesia among doctors in UK hospitals* while others favour brief enigmatic phrases such as *Postlunch dip* or *One-thirty blues*. Others insist on a colon: *Post-lunchtime amnesia: results of a survey*, and a small minority will favour a verb: *More physicians than surgeons doze off after lunch* (Figure 8.3).

Figure 8.3: Characteristics of titles in six journals				
	Active verb	Colon	Fewer than 10 words	20 words or more	Mean no. of words in title (s.d.)
N Engl J Med	14	–	11	1	12.1 (±3.8)
*Lancet**	2	7	9	1	13.4 (±4.1)
*BMJ**	3	33	4	10	16.2 (±4.1)
J Ped	9	12	12	6	13.6 (±4.9)
Ped Research	23	5	7	5	14.3 (±4.3)
*Arch Dis Child**	5	4	26	–	9.8 (±3.5)

*European-based journals.
Source: 50 consecutive articles from June 1, 1997.

Authors should take a pragmatic approach. From their point of view, the good title is one that the editor approves, without changing. Wait until your article is complete before even thinking about writing it. Research your target journal first, then write the title to fit in with this style. The task should take about ten minutes. If (or when) your co-authors start suggesting titles that are clearly unsuitable for your target journal, point out to them gently why your version is more acceptable.

Authors

List the first name, middle initial and last name of each author, with highest academic degree(s) and institutional affiliation.

Also list the name of department(s) and institution(s) to which the work should be attributed. That's the easy part.

In Chapter 3 I warned that authorship was a problem area. As the paper approaches publication you will meet more and more pressure from those who see the small part they played as an opportunity to enhance their CVs. Editors disapprove, but they may seem a distant problem. Be realistic: allow fellow travellers to climb on board if you must, but be careful: if there are too many it might reduce your chances of being published.

You may also find yourself coming under pressure regarding the order in which the authors are to be listed. The Vancouver Group requirements do not really help, stating firmly: 'The order of authorship should be a joint decision of the co-authors. Because the order is assigned in different ways, its meaning cannot be inferred accurately unless it is stated by the authors.' Some journals now require authors to state what they did,[15] which can help to weed out obvious impostors.

Make clear which author is responsible for correspondence about the manuscript and who will be responsible for supplying reprints. Remember that there can be a time-lag between acceptance and publication; make sure that your address will still hold true and warn the editor if, for example, you are taking a temporary post overseas. You don't want to delay an already complex publishing process.

Acknowledgements

It is open to question whether it helps readers or advances knowledge to know that Mrs Antrobus has helped with the library search. But sometimes debts have to be paid. Whenever possible use a technique of expressing thanks that doesn't detract from this method of communicating science – a box of chocolates, perhaps, or a simple thank-you letter.

The Vancouver Group states that this is the place to acknowledge the help of:

- those who have made a contribution, such as 'general support by a departmental chair'
- technical help
- financial and material support
- financial relationships that may pose a conflict of interest (Figure 8.4).

Figure 8.4: The Vancouver Group on acknowledgements

Persons who have contributed intellectually to the paper but whose contributions do not justify authorship may be named and their function or contribution described – for example scientific adviser, critical review of study proposal, data collection or participation in clinical trials. Such persons must have given their permission to be named. Authors are responsible for obtaining written permission from persons acknowledged by name, because readers may infer their endorsement of the data and conclusions.

Technical help should be acknowledged in a paragraph separate from those acknowledging other contributions.

You must declare if there is the slightest reason to suggest that your work may be biased. For instance, if your paper has overwhelmingly discovered that Obecalp is the treatment of choice for post-lunchtime amnesia, you should make it clear that the research was funded by the company that is set to make millions from its use.

A short running header or footer

This should be no more than 40 characters (count letters and spaces) placed at the foot of the title page. It will be used to identify that paper.

The abstract

An abstract can be a stand-alone item of writing (for presenting at conferences, for instance) but in this case it is a summary. Originally it was the final paragraph of the scientific paper. Then it was moved up to the front of the article where it not only attracts attention to that article, but also satisfies that interest without forcing the reader to plough through the text and tables. It is also used as a 'product' on its own, available in abstract journals and on electronic databases. It follows that the abstract should reflect the article accurately. This sounds like an obvious rule, but it is often broken: a recent study found that 18–68% of abstracts in six major journals had data that were inconsistent with, or absent from, the body of the text.[16]

The Vancouver Group gives a clear account of the requirements (Figure 8.5). From the writing point of view, consider this as a separate piece of work. Set yourself a brief (see Chapter 3). The message will be identical to that of the article, as will the market. The length, however, will be different. Once you have set the brief, collect the information, in this case from your article. Do not go back to your original research and do not add any new material.

Figure 8.5: The Vancouver Group on the abstract

The second page should carry an abstract (of no more than 150 words for unstructured abstracts or 250 words for structured abstracts). The abstract should state the purposes of the study or investigation, basic procedures (selection of study subjects or laboratory animals; observational and analytical methods), main findings (giving specific data and their statistical significance, if possible) and the principal conclusions. It should emphasise new and important aspects of the study or observations.

Once you have collected the information, make a plan. Check on the precise guidelines for the preferred structure in the

Instructions to authors, and you can test these by looking at what appears in the journal. If they prefer structured abstracts (Figure 8.6), provide one.

Figure 8.6: Structured abstract

Prevalence of post-lunchtime amnesia among doctors in UK hospitals: results of a cross-sectional survey

Objective: To measure the cumulative prevalence of post-lunchtime amnesia in a representative sample of the consultant population of UK hospitals.

Design: Cross-sectional survey with an anonymous self-administered questionnaire centred on a factual description of post-lunchtime amnesia.

Setting: 68 hospitals randomly selected from 201 hospitals in the UK.

Subjects: 1193 consultants consented to the study and returned completed questionnaires.

Results: 192 (33.8%) physicians and 60 (10.9% surgeons) reported at least one episode of post-lunchtime amnesia in the past four weeks. The prevalence of cases of post-lunchtime amnesia 20.4% (116 cases) among physicians and 3.3% (18) among surgeons.

Conclusions: Post-lunchtime amnesia is a universal phenomenon and could have significant effect on health care. More research is indicated.

When you have your plan, write your abstract in one go. Leave it at least overnight. Then read it again, compare it with your paper, and insert any necessary facts. Adjust the style as required: there is a convention that abstracts are written in the passive voice, and if your target journal favours this style, follow it. This is not the place to campaign for plain English.

After you have written the abstract, pull out some key words (Figure 8.7).

Figure 8.7: The Vancouver Group on key words

Below the abstract authors should provide, and identify as such, 3–10 key words or short phrases that will assist indexers in cross indexing the article and may be published with the abstract. Terms from the medical subject headings (MeSH) list of *Index Medicus* should be used; if suitable MeSH terms are not yet available for recently introduced terms, present terms may be used.

References

Strictly speaking, the references are an integral part of the text and not an additional item. You will already have chosen those papers that you wish to cite, and you will probably have gathered a list of some kind, which may look plausible. But put aside some time to check, double-check and tidy up (Figure 8.8).

Figure 8.8: The Vancouver Group on references

References should be numbered consecutively in the order in which they are first mentioned in the text. Identify references in text, tables, and legends by Arabic numerals in parentheses. References cited only in tables or in legends to figures should be numbered in accordance with the sequence established by the first identification in the text of the particular table or figure . . .

Avoid using abstracts as references. References to papers accepted but not yet published should be designated as in press or forthcoming; authors should obtain written permission to cite such papers as well as verification that they have been accepted for publication. Information from manuscripts submitted but not accepted should be cited in the text as unpublished observations with written permission from the source.

Avoid citing a personal communication unless it provides essential information not available from a public source, in which case the name of the person and date of communication should be cited in parentheses in the text. For scientific articles, authors should obtain written permission and confirmation of accuracy from the source of a personal communication.

The responsibility to get it right is yours. The Vancouver style says: 'The references must be verified by the author(s) against the original documents'. And herein lies a major problem. A study carried out on four dermatology journals in the USA found that, of all the references cited, about one-third could not be traced, one-third did not say what they were said to have said, and only about one-third were accurate.[17] The authors say, with a certain understatement, that this questions the whole business of citing papers.

Check that the papers you cite are doing what they should be doing, which is supporting assertions in the text. If they do not, are you merely engaging in academic name-dropping, which is not what references are for? (Even if you do feel it is politically expedient to cite key papers written by members of the editorial board, at least link them in to the text somehow, and not have then hanging about on their own.)

You should have actually read the papers you cite, and ensured that they say what you say they do. Make sure also that the numbers in the text are the same as the numbers in the list of references, and that there are no discrepancies.

Finally a plea on behalf of professional copy-editors, who say that sorting our references is not only the worst aspect of their job, but also the most time-consuming. Make sure that you follow the style as laid down in the *Instructions to authors*; this doesn't mean simply that the words are roughly in the right order, but that there are not commas where colons should be, and vice versa. Nowadays there is a selection of software that will help you import and collate references, thereby taking out much of the pain that traditionally went with this task. But technology should be in addition to, and not a substitute for, the traditional skill of checking the hard copy yourself.

Tables

You will already have produced your tables and illustrations. Now is the time to check that these are relevant to and enhance readers' understanding of the text. You must also make sure that they meet the criteria for publication and that numbers in tables match those in the text. Prepare the legends: the Vancouver Group gives general guidance (Figure 8.9). Study your target journal's *Instructions to authors* to see if there are any local differences.

Figure 8.9: The Vancouver Group on legends for illustrations

Type or print out legends for illustrations double spaced, starting on a separate page, with Arabic numerals corresponding to the illustrations. When symbols, arrows, numbers, or letters are used to identify parts of the illustrations, identify and explain each one clearly in the legend. Explain the internal scale and identify the method of staining in photomicrographs.

Letter to the editor

This is sometimes considered an afterthought, but don't under-estimate the importance of the letter to the editor. Some editors may say that they don't read them, or pay little attention to them, but, frankly, I don't believe them. It is clear that this is the first thing to come out of the envelope, and therefore it sets the tone for what is to come. A good letter will prepare the way for moving the paper forward for further consideration; a bad letter can hasten rejection (Figures 8.10 and 8.11).

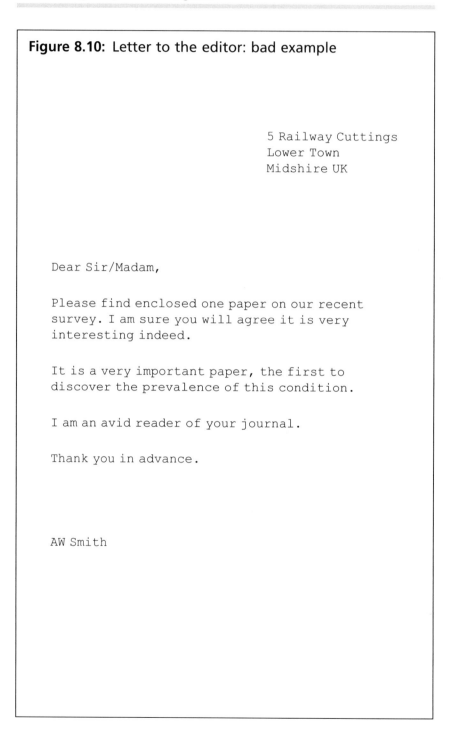

Figure 8.10: Letter to the editor: bad example

5 Railway Cuttings
Lower Town
Midshire UK

Dear Sir/Madam,

Please find enclosed one paper on our recent survey. I am sure you will agree it is very interesting indeed.

It is a very important paper, the first to discover the prevalence of this condition.

I am an avid reader of your journal.

Thank you in advance.

AW Smith

Figure 8.11: Letter to the editor: good example

Department of Amnesia
University of Wherever
Midtown
England KK8 4LL
From the Professor of Prandiology

Dear Professor Jones,

Prevalence of post-lunchtime amnesia among doctors in UK hospitals: results of a cross-sectional survey

I have pleasure in submitting the above paper for your consideration.

In the last 12 months you have published two papers, one of which came from our team, outlining the devastating effect of individual cases of post-lunchtime amnesia. Our results are the first to show the prevalence of this controversial condition.

I confirm that this article has been read and approved by all the co-authors.

Yours sincerely,

AW Smith   WAW Smith   ES Dupont

A good letter will establish three things:

1 who you are
2 what you are submitting
3 why it should be published.

Publishing an article is to some extent a leap of faith by an editor, so establish your credentials as soon as you can. This is achieved as much as by how the letter looks as by the words you use. Use proper headed writing paper. This will establish you as a member of a proper department, and may also give supplementary information, such as department heads, that could strike a positive chord and encourage the editor to trust you.

Lay out the text neatly. Professional communicators have known for some time that the type we use and the way we use it can contribute to whether or not our messages get through. Letters with narrow margins may be seen (unfairly no doubt) to come from people who are unfriendly. Letters with grey type are considered boring. On the other hand those with broad white margins and good black type are considered to be organised and reliable.

Be mindful of the niceties. Address the editor by name, and you can easily find this by looking at the publication details. Do not insult the editor by spelling his or her name or title wrong.

Put the title of the paper at the top of your letter. But also explain it in the text, making sure that you use a verb, so that the editor knows what the message is, and not just the subject matter. It will also help your case if you can state tactfully why it should be published. Do not be rude, and say that it's about time the editor published something good. Do not be cute: editors will not be impressed by the fact that you have long enjoyed their journal. Do not offer a bribe. But you can point out that, for instance, the journal has been running a number of articles on this subject and your paper offers an elegant solution to the debate.

Take note of any special demands in the *Instructions to authors*. If required (and it usually is), make sure that all authors sign the covering letter. If the journal requires that you need to sign over the copyright, make clear your assent. Nothing irritates an editor more than having to chase up details that should have been supplied before. It takes time away from other things, but also raises the question: if this person can't read the *Instructions to authors*, how much value should be given to his researches proper?

Before proceeding to Chapter 9, you should have:
- written all the additional items that go with a scientific article
- prepared a positive letter to the editor.

BOOKCHOICE: Checking the details

Fraser J (1997) *How to Publish in Biomedicine*. Radcliffe Medical Press, Oxford.
Byrne DW (1998) *Publishing Your Medical Research Paper*. Williams & Wilkins, Baltimore.

Throughout my book I take the view that the best way to write something is to 'think big' – take risks, write with broad strokes, and ignore the multiple obstacles that seem to be put in your way. But there comes a stage when the need for this type of creativity starts drawing to a close, and you must start the painstaking work of checking, double-checking and polishing. For this I suggest taking advantage of the current trend for publishing books that deal with their subject in a succession of heavily signposted checklists.

Jane Fraser, in a book which comes from the UK–European tradition, offers 216 pages with '500 tips for success' ranging from a section-by-section guide to research papers to clear writing and useful websites. It is packed with information: the 31 tips about tables, for instance, are followed by an 11-point 'reviewer's checklist': 'Do the tables match journal style . . . each deal with a specific question . . . etc?' As she writes, the book 'is intended to answer the commonest questions about scientific writing, and to help you avoid the most frequent problems and pitfalls'.

Daniel Byrne, who belongs to the US tradition, offers more pages (298) but fewer tips (200). He covers much the same ground, but has a glitzier approach and includes some new research on what reviewers think. For instance, they say that the most common reasons for rejecting a paper outright are inadequate or inappropriate presentation of data and failure to give a detailed explanation of the design. However, what reviewers and editors say is not necessarily what they choose: for reasons stated in my book I would urge writers to ignore, for instance, principle 83 which urges authors to think of a snappy title, or principle 88 which urges writers of the introduction to 'start with thunder'.

One word of warning: reading this kind of book can be a marvellous way of not actually getting down to the writing. I advise that you do not refer to these until after the first draft.

9

Use internal reviewers

'Many people find reviewers' comments difficult to handle. I don't, so long as I think they're reasonable, but when reviewers disagree with each other, it's a problem.'

'Hit me again . . . and again . . .'

This may be one of the shortest chapters in this book, but it deals with the process that is often the longest and most painful. You will have sweated over your statistics, selected from half a mile of references, and agonised over the exact phrasing for a dozen difficult concepts. Now, as you bring your beautiful baby into the world, people are about to tear it limb from limb. And these are the people who are meant to be your friends.

Remain focused on your goal: you want to be a published author. Good advice from other people will be invaluable, essential even. However, much of the advice you get will not necessarily be good, and may even reduce your chances of becoming published. How do you handle this?

One step forward is to divide this process of internal reviewing into two stages: voluntary and compulsory

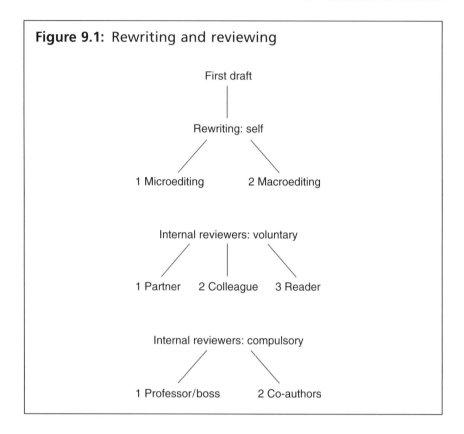

Figure 9.1: Rewriting and reviewing

First draft

Rewriting: self

1 Microediting   2 Macroediting

Internal reviewers: voluntary

1 Partner   2 Colleague   3 Reader

Internal reviewers: compulsory

1 Professor/boss   2 Co-authors

(Figure 9.1). During the voluntary stage you should choose those whose opinions you value and invite their comments in a structured way. You remain free to choose those comments with which you agree. The compulsory stage can come later, and involves showing your manuscript to those whose opinions you are less free to discard. These are co-authors and 'bosses'. Your role is to hear what they have to say, accept it when they have something to contribute, but negotiate when they are trying to impose changes that, in your view, are going to decrease the chances of becoming published. The second stage, therefore, is more about negotiating skills than writing techniques.

Voluntary reviewing

One of the reasons that this stage can become so unpleasant is the way we approach it. We send off our article to a number of colleagues with a brief note saying 'Any comments?'. This is asking for trouble: the only way they can fail in this task is to say nothing. So they make dozens of pencil marks, each of which sears into your soul as a sign of your inadequacy and lack of education.

Choose carefully who you will invite and why. You will probably need four different types of feedback, and therefore you should choose at least one person for each question. When you ask for their help, be specific about what you want them to do.

To an outsider: can you spot any stupid mistakes?

We all make basic errors, such as: 'The doctors did all they could to elevate the discomfort'. We therefore need someone with common sense, plus the motivation to catch us out. Partners do this task particularly well. This can be deeply distressing for authors, who have to face the evidence of their fallibility, but it is worth it.

To a linguist: is the language appropriate?

If English is not your first language, consider asking someone to look over your article for style. There are various views on whom you should ask. Some say you should choose a professional linguist, such as someone who has studied at university. The danger is that they may be slightly out of touch with modern idioms, and I recommend instead someone who still listens to the BBC. You need someone to be able to point out that the following aren't quite right:

- she was cycling from Menarche onwards
- the apparent islands are in reality branches of a richly arborising tree-like structure.

Keep it in perspective, however. As Bill Whimster has written: 'I believe that editors will not be prejudiced against a [poorly written] paper unless they cannot understand what the author means or unless the paper is already borderline in terms of its message and proof, originality, importance or suitability for the journal'.[18]

To a colleague: are there any major omissions or logical flaws?

Try to avoid at this stage showing your manuscript to the world's greatest living expert on your subject. You will almost certainly fall off their agenda, which is to show you that they are the world's greatest living expert. At this stage you need someone with a similar level of knowledge to yours who can point to any major gaps that may have occurred, such as a fault of logic in your argument or a major paper you have missed.

To another colleague: if you were the reviewer what would you say?

Find someone who is typical of your target audience, by which I mean the journal's editor and reviewers rather than its readers. If you know someone who has done any reviewing, ask them how they would react if they were sent this paper.

Compulsory reviewing

Now you must play a completely different game. This is the compulsory internal reviewing, in which negotiation skills become a vital tool.

Co-authors can cause trouble. At their worst, they will have wanted you to have written a different article. As suggested in Chapter 3, one way of reducing this kind of dispute is to make sure that, at an early stage, all co-authors agree with your brief. At least then you have some common ground on which to fall back.

Even if you can get them to agree over the article's message and market, co-authors will quibble about the style. This can be tiresome. It can also be dangerous when they insist, for instance, that you adopt a certain style that you know from your market research is not suited to your target journal. Your only recourse is to show them your evidence, and argue your point with as little emotion as possible.

Then there are professors. What do you do with those who, after you have carefully researched your market and noticed that it prefers to use short words and the active voice, carefully change it all back again on the grounds that you are not writing scientifically? In principle, it is better to negotiate than it is to argue or to sulk. Point out what the style of the journal happens to be, and back it up with evidence from that journal. You may not win the argument, but at least you will have tried. (And when you become a professor, you can remember not to fall into the same trap.)

You are unlikely to win every battle. If you are the first author, then in theory the decision is yours, though that becomes academic (if you will pardon the pun) if you are a very junior doctor and your critic is a very senior professor. At this stage we are really talking about damage limitation.

Before proceeding to Chapter 10 you should have:
- improved your manuscript by taking into account the best comments from a wide range of people
- prevented others from making it unpublishable.

BOOKCHOICE: Taking advice from professionals

Winokur J (ed) (1999) *Advice to Writers*. Pantheon Books, New York.

If you have got this far you can start calling yourself a writer. So treat yourself to this book, which will amuse you and help you to improve your writing at the same time. Author Jon Winokur has combed autobiographies, diaries, letters and books to come up with more than 400 bits of advice by writers for writers, arranged in 36 sections from agents and characters to the writer's life and writing advice.

Some of it, such as the sections on agents and dialogue, will not be relevant to the writing of scientific papers – but much of it will be. On general matters, be consoled by John Berryman on reacting to criticism: 'I would recommend the cultivation of extreme indifference to both praise and blame because praise will lead you to vanity, and blame will lead you to self pity, and both are bad for writers'. Consider James Thurber's 'Don't get it right, get it written' or TS Eliot's 'Whatever you do . . . avoid piles'.

There's good advice on style that will come in useful at this stage. 'A good style must first of all, be clear. It must not be mean or above the dignity of the subject. It must be appropriate' (Aristotle). 'When you say something make sure you have said it. The chances of your having said it are only fair' (EB White). Or 'Read over your compositions and when you meet a passage which you think is particularly fine, strike it out' (Samuel Johnson).

There's also some advice on specifics that backs up many of the points made in this book: 'Short words are best and the old words when short are best of all' (Winston Churchill) or 'You should not take hyphens seriously' (Sir Ernest Gowers).

10

Send off the package

'It will have to go. There's work waiting to be done.'

At last . . .

Assemble the package. Keep a copy of everything you send: work on the principle that, in the world of publishing, anything that can get mislaid will get mislaid. Make one last check (Figure 10.1), put all the elements in a sound envelope, double-check you have the right address, put on a stamp – and put it in the post.

As soon as you do this you will be desperate to know whether 'They' like it. This is a difficult time, and a sensible solution is to go on holiday, preferably on a small boat with no mobile telephone.

. . . into the black hole

If the journal staff is well organised, you should hear from them within a few days. Unfortunately they will only tell you whether your paper has arrived, and not whether they are going to publish it or not.

Figure 10.1: Final checklist

- Submission letter, signed by all authors
- Original and copies of article

  Title page

  Abstract

  Article

  References

  Tables

  Legends
- Sets of illustrations, properly labelled
- Patient consent letters or permission to reproduce previously published material
- Copyright agreement.

If after about three weeks you have not even received an acknowledgement, it is quite acceptable to telephone with an enquiry. Do not ask to speak to the editor. He or she will probably not have the slightest idea who you are or whether your precious manuscript has arrived. Instead ring the editor's secretary or an editorial assistant who will probably have the day-to-day responsibility for logging copy in and out. Don't be hostile: ask simply to confirm whether or not the paper has arrived.

Over the next few weeks it will seem that your magnificent creation has disappeared into a large black hole. But because you can't see any action, it doesn't mean that your manuscript is being neglected. A sophisticated (and usually well-oiled) procedure is now swinging into action to receive and assess it. Retain a sense of proportion: your paper represents months of work for you, but for the staff it is almost certainly one of several that arrived that day. The *BMJ*, for example, receives on average more than 20 papers each working day, which is also good reason for a brief but convincing covering letter.

Editors go to enormous lengths to ensure that the system gives authors a fair hearing. If you have sent your article to one of the larger, general journals, it will probably be dealt with by a medically qualified assistant editor. He or she will read your article, and make a decision whether to send it straight back as perfectly hopeless, or whether to progress it through the system. The good news is that if you don't get it back immediately you have passed the first hurdle.

Your manuscript will then go forward to two reviewers. They will make their assessment and return the manuscript, which could at this stage be sent back to the author, either as a straight rejection or with a recommendation to make some major changes and resubmit. The journal will then hold a selection meeting, which may include practising doctors among the assessors. (At the *BMJ* this is pretentiously called the hanging committee, after the Royal Academy.) Editors handling each paper will make a presentation, and there will be some haggling. In general the meeting will agree, but the editor has the right to overrule all this advice. As shown in Chapter 1, his or her responsibilities are broader than to an individual author. The systems on a specialist journal are similar.

Coping with rejection

Rare is the author who has not been rejected. When it happens to you, be as mature as possible. Dry your eyes, leave the rejection letter for a couple of days, then start your post-mortem.

You may wish to blame your rejection on the nature of the reviewing system, but that is a fruitless exercise. You should take responsibility for the failure, though you will find it helpful to ask 'Why did my marketing not succeed this time?' rather than 'Why did I fail?'.

One advantage of the reviewing system is that you will usually be told the reasons for rejection. Are the criticisms fair? Can you answer them? Should you consider an appeal? You should certainly *not* appeal if the letter says something like 'We enjoyed reading your article but we do not feel it is a priority for us at the moment . . .' Reading carefully between the lines will show you that this is a value judgement. The only grounds of appeal would be that you know the editor's job better than he or she. This approach is not likely to win friends and secure publication.

On the other hand, you may feel – and may even be justified in feeling – that the reviewers have misinterpreted what you have said. In this case you have every right to appeal, but do so politely. Do not write and berate the editor for choosing such idiots for reviewers. Do write a considered and polite letter, setting out clearly where you disagree with the reviewers – and what your evidence is. Sometimes your appeal will be upheld.

Another, and more common, alternative is to submit your article elsewhere. Do not simply print out your covering letter again, deleting all references to the editor of the *New England Journal* and substituting the name of the editor of the *Transylvanian Annals of Left Handed Surgery*. Re-examine your product carefully. What is your new market and does your message still hold for it? In other words, go back to Chapter 3 and start again. The process should be far quicker this time. Be encouraged by the fact that most rejected papers eventually get published.

Throughout your dealings with editors and reviewers, do as you would be done by. It's a bit like the doctor–patient relationship, though this time you are the patient. There are striking similarities between a nightmare patient and a nightmare writer: refusal to admit error, persistency, reluctance to take advice.

Of course, there comes a time in every task when we have to realise that it won't succeed. But when do you know when to stop submitting? The answer is relatively straightforward. When you start getting the same kind of objections from the reviewers and you are unable to meet them, then you should call it a day. And channel your energies into another paper.

Coping with acceptance

So much for the gloom. There will almost certainly come a time when you reach the promised land and find that an article you have written has been accepted. This is likely to be a qualified acceptance, if only because editors and reviewers feel that they are failing in their job if they don't criticise. But there will be a clear implication – even a firm promise – that they will publish your paper provided you make the recommended changes. Make sure that you do these changes as quickly as possible. I often meet people who have interpreted a qualified acceptance as a rejection, thereby missing out on the chance of publication.

You can start to rejoice as your article moves towards the process of publication. But even at this stage there are one or two pitfalls lying ahead.

Be careful of prior publication. Some journals will not publish anything that has been published elsewhere. The nightmare scenario is that your paper is being prepared for publication, and at the same time you are giving a presentation to a conference. There present an astute reporter from a lay paper, who recognises the important implications of what you have done – and, as his job requires him to do, writes it up accordingly. In theory, your paper, though accepted, could now be rejected. The best way of dealing with this is to liaise in advance with the editor. Let him or her know what is happening, and there should be no problems.

You should soon receive a proof of your article. Do not be

surprised if it differs from your version. That is because all publications have someone – either professional or part-time – whose job it is to copy-edit all articles. They will carry through a number of checks. They will – if they have time, which most of them increasingly say they have not – carry out some stylistic changes in order to make your article more suitable for their target audience.

Trust their judgement; they will normally have considerable experience at their job, plus detailed knowledge of the demands of their readership. Do not be over-proprietorial with what you have written and under no circumstances should you reinstate your version word for word.

On the other hand, do not just tick the proof without reading it. Check it carefully for accuracy. Look for the obvious spelling mistakes. Check the numbers. Look at dosages and check names and titles. Make sure you meet any deadlines.

After publication

Now is the time to forget the pain. You are about to become a Published Author. Enjoy the experience. You will have earned it.

Take a short rest, then work out whether you want to get back to healing the sick – or start all over again.

If you have got this far, you should have become a published author. Celebrate. And recommend this book to a friend.

References

1 Lock S (ed) (1991) *The Future of Medical Journals*. BMJ Publications, London.

2 Court C and Dillner L (1994) Obstetrician suspended after research inquiry. *BMJ*. **309**: 1459.

3 Altman LK (1996) The Ingelfinger rule, embargoes and journal peer review, Part 2. *Lancet*. **347**: 1459–63.

4 Klauser HA (1987) *Writing on Both Sides of The Brain*. HarperCollins, San Francisco.

5 *Journal Citation Reports* (1995) Institute for Scientific Information Inc, Philadelphia.

6 Annals of Internal Medicine (1997) *Uniform Requirements for Manuscripts Submitted to Biomedical Journals* (5e). American College of Physicians, Philadelphia. Single copies are available free of charge from the URM Secretariat Office, American College of Physicians, Independence Mall West, Sixth Street at Race, Philadelphia, 19106-1572, USA. Correspondence to Kathleen Case: Tel: 00 1 215 351 2661; Fax: 00 1 215 351 2644; email: mhs:kathyc@acp The requirements are not covered by copyright and may therefore be copied or reprinted without permission if such use is not for profit.

7 Buzan T and Buzan B (1993) *The Mind Map Book*. BBC Books, London.

8 Gunning R (1971) *The Technique of Clear Writing*. McGraw Hill, New York.

9 Altman DG (1996) Better reporting of randomised controlled trials: the CONSORT statement. *BMJ*. **313**: 570–1.

10 Howard G (1993) *The Good English Guide*. Pan Macmillan, Basingstoke.

11 Gowers E (1996) *The Complete Plain Words* (3e). (Revised by Greenbaum S and Whitcut J) The Stationery Office, London.

12 The Lancet (1937) *On Writing for The Lancet*. Supplement to edition of 2.1.37.

13 Matthews JR, Bowen JM and Matthews RW (1996) *Successful Scientific Writing*. Cambridge University Press, Cambridge.

14 Smith R (1996) In: *Short Words* (newsletter of TAA Training). TAA Training, Leatherhead.

15 Smith R (1997) Authorship is dying: long live contributorship. *BMJ*. **315**: 696.

16 Pitkin RM, Branagen MA and Burmeister LF (1999) Accuracy of data in abstracts of published research articles. *JAMA*. **281**(12): 1110–11.

17 George PM and Robbins K (1994) Reference accuracy in the dermatologic literature. *J Am Acad Dermatol*. **31**(i): 61–4.

18 Whimster WF (1997) *Biomedical Research: how to plan, publish and present it*. Springer-Verlag, London.

Index